Treatments of
Gastrorantestranal Diseases
in Traditional Chinese Medicine

Chief-editor   Hou Jinglun   Zhao Xin

Academy Press [Xue Yuan]

First Edition 1995

ISBN7-5077-0770-9/R · 128

Treatments of Gastrorantestranal Diseases in Traditional Chinese Medicine

Chief-Editor   Hou Jinglun   Zhao Xin

Published by Academy Press [Xue yuan]

Distributed by

China International Book Trading Corporation

35 Chegongzhuang Xilu, Beijing 100044, China

P. O. Box 399, Beijing, China

Printed in the People's Republic of China

Introduction to
Collections of Traditional Chinese Medicine

Traditional Chinese Medicine and Pharmacology(TCMP) has a long history. TCMP summed up abundant clinical experience in the struggle against diseases. It has formed an integrated, unique and first of all, a scientific system of both theory and clinical practice. On the fundamental principle of "Zhengtiguannian"(Wholism) and "Bian-Zhenglunzhi"(Treatment of the same disease with different therapies), TCM treatment is effective for various kind of diseases with few side-effect taken. At present, a great upsurge in learning, practising and studying TCM is just in the accendant. For the benefit of people of all countries, we compiled this series of "Collections of Traditional Chinese Medicine" in order to promote the spread of TCM all over the world. The collections includes: Traditional Chinese Treatment for Cardiovascular diseases. Traditional Chinese Treatment for Respiratory Diseases. Traditional Chinese Medicine in Gastroenterology etc.

In these books, we introduced comprehensively TCM treatment for commonly encountered diseases and therapies such as drug therapy, acupuncture and moxibustion, Qigong, massage, dietic therapy, etc. are suggested accordingly. This series is the best for these foreign friends who want to learn and master TCM.

May everyone of all nations enjoy a healthy life!

Chief-Editor
Hou Jinglun

CONTENTS

Chapter One   Chronic Gastritis

Chapter Two   Gastroduodenal Ulcers

Chapter Three   Viral Hepatitis

Chapter Four   Chronic Hepatitis

Chapter Five   Hepatocirrhosis

Chapter Six Cholecystitis

Chapter Seven Ulcerative Colitis

Chapter Eight Constipation

Chapter Nine   Diarrhea

Chapter Ten   Spasm of Diaphragm

Chapter Eleven   Infantile Anorexia

Chapter Twelve Epidemic Parotitis

Chapter Thirteen Bacillary Dysentery

Chapter Fourteen Carcinoma of Esophagus

Chapter Fifteen   Carcinoma of Stomach

Chapter Sixteen Recipes for Treating Disorders of Digestive System

Chapter One
Chronic Gastritis

Chronic gastritis is a chronic gastric lesion, pathologically characterized by nonspecific chronic inflammation of the gastric mucosa. Its etiology is not well understood, possibly related to administration of irritating drugs and food, bile regurgitation, buccal inflammation or autoimmunity. Chronic gastritis can be divided into two categories, primary and secondary. The former is further categorized into superficial , atrophic and hypertrophic types; the latter often complicates gastroduodenal ulcrt and gastric cancer.

Histologically, when inflammatory cells (neutrophils, lymphocytes, plasma cells, and a few cosinophils) are limited to the gastric pits and upper lamina propria, gastritis is classified as superficial. In atrophic gastritis, inflammatory cells invade deeper into the lamina propria and glandular epithelim. Lymphoid follicles may also be seen. As the disease progresses, thinning of the mucosa occurs with loss of glandular elements. In some patients intestinal metaplasia develops with loss of parietal and chief cells and development of goblet cells, absorptive cells, and intestinal willi. Finally, in patients with gastric atrophy, parietal and chief cells are absent, mucosal thickness is reduced markedly, and only a small number of inflammatory cells are present.

Chronic atrophuy gastritis has been divided into Type A and type B, based primarily on the anatomic portion of the stomach involved and the presence or absence of parietal cell antibodies. In Type A gastritis, the fundus and body of the stomach are involved, whereas the antrum is relatively normal. Parietal cell antibodies are found in a large percentage of patients, and pernicious anemia may develop. On the other hand, in Type B gastritis the antrum is involved primarily. Although inflammation is found frequently in the fundus and body, parietal cell antibodies do not occur.

In traditional Chinese medicine, there is no equivalent term for chronic gastritis and this condition is described as disharmony of the function and coordination of the liver and stomach, due to stagnation of dampness caused by deficiency of the spleen. This disease pertains to the categories of "pi"(feeling of fullness in the upper abdomen), "wei wan tong" (stomachache), etc.

I ETIOLOGY AND PATHOGENESIS

The following pathogenic factors cause epigastric pain:

① Impairment of the spleen and stomach by improper diet

Irregular food intake, overeating or hunger, as well as ingestion of unclean, decayed and poisonous food, can all impair the qi of both the spleen and stomach. Improper diet includes overindulgence in raw or cold food that causes pathogenic cold to accumulate and both qi and blood to stagnate in the stomach, and consumption of too much greasy food or alcoholic drink that produces damp-heat in the spleen and stomach. These pathogenic factors disturb stomach qi, which fails to descend, resulting in its stagnation, and hence epigastric pain. The etiology and pathogenesis of acute gastritis usually falls under this category.

② Affection of the stomach by hyperactive liver qi

Anxiety, anger and mental depression injure the liver, causing liver qi to stagnate, which affects the normal function of the stomach and the descending of stomach qi, resulting in stomachache. This morbid state is usually called " incoordination between the liver and the stomach". If the liver qi remains depressed for a long time, it may turn to heat, which will consume stomach yin., producing the syndrome of stomach yin deficiency. ％ 3. Deficiency cold of the spleen and stomach

Pathogenic factors, such as overstrain and stress, prolonged illness and improper medical treatment, as well as a congenital defect in the yang of both the spleen and stomach cause this morbid state. These pathogenic factors damage the transporting and transforming functions of the spleen and the descending function of the stomach, resulting in accumulation of pathogeinc damjp in the spleen and stomach, and hence epigastric pain.

Generally speaking, the etiology and pathogenesis of chronic gastritis usually falls under the latter two categories.

II CLINICAL MANIFESTATIONS

The vast majority of persons with chronic gastritis do not have symptoms. Gastrointestinal symptoms, if they Occure, may include anorexia, epigastric pressure and fullness, heartburn, nausea, vomiting, specific food intolerance, a peptic ulcer-like syndrome, and anemia or gross hemorrhage. Physical findings are often absent or consist only of mild epigastric tenderness.

III MAIN POINTS OF DIAGNOSIS

1. The chief symptoms are chronic upper abdominal pain, fullness and discomfort, belching and acid regurgitation which often occur after meals. Mild hemorrhage of upper digestive tract may be induced by some precipitating factors in a few cases. Severe atrophic gastritis may be accompanied with anemia and pathologic leanness.

2. Physical examination reveals mild but diffuse tenderness in the upper abdominal region.

3. Laboratory examination

(1) Gastric juice analysis: Gastric acid is normal in superficial gastritis, but mostly reduced or gone in atrophic gastritis.

(2) X-ray barium examination: Positive rate is not high. Atrophic gastritis presents gastric hypotension, triviality or disappearance of gastric mucosal folds. The main purpose of radiological examination is to exclude peptic ulcer and cancer.

(3) Gastrofiberscope: This method is most contributive in confirming diagnosis. Through it superficial mucosal erosion with hyperemia, swelling or red spots and increased ropy liquid could be discovered in chronic superficial gastritis; in chronic atrophic gastritis, such findings can be caught as thinned and greyish-pale mucosa, slenderized mucosal folds with exposure of submucosal vessels, and granular or nodular proliferation. The combined application of gastrofiberscope and biopsy proves to be an accurate method for the diagnosis of chronic gastritis.

IV DIFFERENTIATION AND TREATMENT OF COMMON SYNDROMES

1. Stagnation of the stomach-qi

Main symptoms and signs: Epigastric distension and fullness or pain, loss of appetite, indigestion, or diarrhea, white coating of the tongue, and slippery pulse.

Therapeutic principle: Regulating the stomach-qi to relieve distension and fullness.

Recipe: Pinellia Decoction for Purging Stomach-fire.

Rhizoma Pinelliae	9g
Rhizoma Zingiberis	9g
Radix Scutellariae	9g
Rhizoma Coptidis	6g
Radix Codonopsis Pilosulae	12g
Rhizoma Glycyrrhizae	9g
Fructus Ziziphi Jujubae	12 pieces

All the above drugs are to be decocted in water for oral administration.

For the case of a more severe stomachache, 15 grams of white peony root (Rhizoma Paeoniae Alba) and 9 grams of corydalis tuber (Rhizoma Corydalis) may be employed.

2. Hyperactive liver-qi attacking the stomach

Main symotoms and signs: Epigastric distension, pain, fullness, oppression and discomfort which is aggravated after meals, frequent belching which may be aggravated by emotional upset, thin and white coating of the tongue, and deep taut pulse.

Therapeutic principle: Relieving hyperactive liver-qi and regulating the stomach.

Recipe: Modified Bupleurum Powder for Relieving Liver-qi.

Radix Bupleuri	10g
Rhizoma Cyperi	10g
Radix Paeoniae Alba	10g
Fructus Aurantii	10g

Fructus Meliae Toosendan	10g
Rhizoma Corydalis	10g
Pericarpium Citri Reticulatae	10g
Caulis Perillae	10g
Radix Glycyrrhizae	6g

All the above drugs are to be decocted in water for oral administration.

If there are acid regurgitation, burning sensation and distresss in the stomach, 15 grams of dandelion herb (Herba Taraxaci), 9 grams of coptis rhizome (Rhizoma Coptidis) and 6 grams of evodia fruit (Fructus Evodiae) are to be added to the recipe.

3. Insufficiency-cold of the spleen and stomach

Main symptoms and sings: Vague pain in the stomach, vomiting of watery fluid, preference for warmth and press, aggravation from cold, mental fatigue and weakness, loose stools, pale tongue, deep thready and weak pulse.

Therapeutic principle: Warming middle-jiao and ispelling pathogenic cold.

Recipe: Modified Decoction of Astragalus for Tonifying Middle-jiao.

Radix Astragali seu Heaysari	30g
Ramulus Cinnamomi	9g
Radix Paeoniae Alba	18g
Radix Aucklandiae	9g
Rhhizoma Zingiberis	6g
Fructus Amomi	10g
Fructus Ziziphi Fujubae	5 pieces
Radix Glycyrrhizae Praeparata	6g

All the above drugs are to be decocted in water for oral administration.

If the case is complicated with anorexia and belching with fetid odour, 10 grams of medicated leaven (Massa Fermentata Medicinalis) and 10 grams of germinated barley (Fructus Hordei Germinatus) may be administered; if the case with acid regurgitation, 30 grams of calcined ark shell(Concha Arcae) added; if the case with dominant cold of insufficiency type, 10 grams of dangshen(Radix Codonopsis Pilosulae), 10 grams of white atractylodes rhizome (Rhizoma Atractylodis Macrocephalae) and 10 grams of poria(Poria) included.

4. Deficiency of the stomach-yin due to stomach-heat

Main symptoms and signs: Irregular stomachache with burning sensation which is aggravated in the afternoon or on empty stomach and is relieved after meals, dry mouth and throat, or thirst, loss of appetite, dry stool, red tongue with yellowish and dty fur, and taut and thready or rapid pulse.

Therapeutic principle: Clearing away heat from the stomach and nourishing the stomach-yin.

Ricipe: Modified Decoction for Nourishing the Stomach.

Radix Glehniae	10g
Radix Ophiopogonis	10g
Rhizoma Polygonati Odorati	10g
Radix Paeoniae Alba	10g
Radix scutellariae	10g
Rhizoma Coptidis	10g
Rhizoma Anemarrhenae	10g
Pericarpium Citri Reticulatae	10g
Herba Taraxaci	20g
Radix glycyrrhizae	6g

All the above drugs are to be decocted in water for oral administration.

5. Blood stasis in the collaterals

Principle of treatment: Promote blood circulation and eliminate blood stasis; it is necessary to determine whether the blood stasis is cansed by qi stagnation or qi deficiency; in the former type, the principle of treatment is to regulate the flow of qi and to remove the blood in order to relieve pain; the latter type should be treated with drugs that replenish qi and promote blood circulation.

Formula of choice:

1) Si Ni San (Powder for treating cold Limbs) or Shi xiao San (Wonderful Powder for Relieving Blood Stagnation) in cases of blood stasis caused by qi stagnation; in these formulae Radix Bupleuri and Fructus Aurantii Immaturus adjust liver qi, and Radix Paeoniae Alba, Pollen Typhae and Faeces Trogopterorum promote blood circulation and remove blood stasis.

2) Liang Fu Wan (Galangal and Cyperus Pill) in addition to Decoction of Invigorating Yang for Recuperation in cases of blood stasis caused by qi deficiency; in this formula Radix Astragali is the Principal ingredient for invigorating qi, Rhizoma Galangae and Rhizoma Cyperus warm the stomach and regulate qi and the other ingredients remove blood stasis.

V ACCUPUNCTRUE AND MOXIBUSTION

①. Principal acupoints: Zhongwan (RN 12), Neiguan (PC 6) and Zusanli (ST 36); Zusanli (ST 36) is the He (sea) Point of the Stomach Meridian, and Zhongwan (RN 12) is the Front-Mu point; these two points used together pacify the stomach and activate the descent of qi; Neiguan (PC 6) is one of the pair-points of the Eight Confluent points and relieves the fullness of the stomach.

Supplementary points:

1) For accumulation of cold and retention of food in the stomach, add shangwan (RN 13) and Pishu (BL 20) to eliminate cold and undigested food.

② If the stomach is attacked by hyperactive liver qi, add Qimen (LR 14) and Taichong (LR 3) to remove stagnated liver qi, regulate its flow and relieve pain.

3) For deficiency cold of the spleen and stomach, apply acupuncture and moxibustion to Qihai (RN 6), Pishu (BL 20), gongsun (SP 4) and Zhangmen (LR 13) to warm the spleen and stomach, eliminate cold, regulate the flow of qi and relieve pain.

4) For blood stasis in collaterals, add Geshu (BL 17), Ganshu (BL 18) and Pishu (BL 20) to regulate the flow of qi and promote blood circulation.

5) For yin deficiency of the spleen and stomach, add Pishu (BL 20), Weishu (BL 21), Sanyinjiao (SP 6) and Taixi (KI 3) to nourish yin and clear away heat from the stomach.

2. Main points: Zhongwan (EN 12), Neiguan (PC 6), Zusanli (ST36) and Weishu (BL21).

Supplementary points: Tianshu (ST 25)) and Quchi (RN 6) for abdominal distention; Pishu (BL20) for indigestion.

Method: 3 or 4 of the main points are punctured with moderate stimulation. the auxiliary points are prescribed according to the symptoms. the needles are retained for 15 minutes and the therapy is given once daily.

3. Principal acupoints: Neiguan (PC 6), Zhongwan (RN 12) and Zusanli (ST 36).

Supplementary points: For deficiency cold in the spleen and stomach, Pishu

(BL 20), Weishu (BL 21) and Gongsun (SP 4) are added; for attack of the stomach by the liver-qi, Yanglingquan (GB 34), Taichong (LR 3) and Qimen (LR 14) ; for stagnancy of qi and blood stasis, Ganshu (BL 18), Geshu (BL 17) and Sanyinjiao (SP 6).

Method: For attack of the stomach by the liver-qi and stagnancy of qi and blood stasis, the even movement or reducing method may be used; for deficdiency-cold in the spleen and stomach, the reinforcing method kis adopted, and moxibustion is added.

4. Ear-acupuncture therapy

1) Points: Stomach Pt, Spleen Pt Liver Pt Sympathetic Nerve Pt and Shenmen Pt.

Method: All the above points are punctured once daily with moderate stimulation and the needles are retained for 30 to 60 minutes.

2) Prescription: Pt, Liver, Pt, Stomach, Pt. Sympathetic Nerve, and Pt, Subcortes.

Method: 2-3 points are selected for each treatment.

Retain the needles for 15-30 minutes. The auricular-seed-pressing therapy is also applicable.

5. Point injection therapy

Points: Weishu(BL21), Pishu(BL20), Ganshu(BL18), Zhongwan(RN 12), Liangmen(ST21). Zusanli(ST36) and Sanyinjiao(SP6).

Drugs: Vitamin B.

Method: Each time 3 or 4 of the above points are injected with 0. 5 to 1 millilitre of the above drug in each. The therapy is given once daily.

IV MASSAGE

This disease needs a long course of treatment with a massage therapy. It should be distinguished from gastritic cancer, gastritic ulcer and duodenal ulcer. In the course of treatment, the patient should avoid taking gastric mucosa-stimulating medicines, cultivate a good habit of diet and a good way of life, and avoid eating excess-cold and pungent food.

1. Manipulation : Pushing with one-finger meditation, rubbing, pressing

kneading, obliquely-pulling, etc.

2. Location of points: Zhongwan (RN 12), Qihai (RN 6), Neiguan (PC 6), Pishu (BL 20), Weishu (BL 21), Ganshu (BL 18), Zusanli (ST 36), etc.

3. Operation

1) The patient is in supine position with upper limbs naturally put at two sides of the body respectively and the hip and knee slightly flexed. The doctor rubs with palm the upper abdomen (a little bit to the left) clockwise for 300-500 times.

Talc powder may be used as a medium and the manipulation should be light, soft and continuous.

2) The posture is the same as the mentioned above. the doctor pushes with one finger from Zhongwan (RN 12) upwards to Shangwan (RN 13). The pushing should be slow and last for 3-5 minutes.

3) With the middle finger, the doctor vibrates Zhongwan (RN 12) for 3-5 minutes.

4) The doctor press-kneads Qihai (RN 6) with the thumb or the middle finger for 2-3 minutes.

5) The patient is in supine position, mwith lower limbsstretched straight, relaxes the whole body and the doctor press-kneads Zusanli (ST 36) with the thumb for 3-5 minutes.

6) The patient is in prone position, the waist and back revealed and coated with Chineses holly leaf. The doctor, standing to his right, scrubs the lateral parts of the spine and waist with right palm or minor thenar eminance focusing on Pishu (BL 20) and Weishu (BL 21), till the heat produced penetrates the abdomen, and then with empty palm lightly pats the lower chest and upper waist for 5-10 minutes.

7) The operator stands behind the sitting patient, grasps Jianjing (GB 21) with two hands, press-kneads Shousanli (LI 10), Neiguan (PC 6) and Hegu (LI 4) of the upper limbs in an orderly way, 30-50 times for each point; then foulages and shakes upper limbs; finally foulage-rubs costal regions from above to below for 3-5 times.

4. Modification of Manipulation according to Different Syndromes

1) In the case of a dull pain in gastric cavity, joy for hot and pressing, anorexia, gastric distension and fullness after meal, sallow complexion and weak-

ness, which is called dificiency of qi of the spleen and stomach, also press-knead Pishu (BL 20), Weishu (BL 21), Zhangmen (LR 13) and Neiguan (PC 6).

2) In the case of distending pain, fullness and discomfort in the tomach especially after meals, wandering pain radiating to hypochondria and aggravated by emotional upset, frequent eructation, relieved when there is wind from bowels, acid regurgitation and vomitus, which is called stagnation of qi of liver and stomach, also press-knead Qimen (LR 14), Ganshu (BL 18), Yanglingquan (GB 34) and Taichong (LR 3).

3) In the case of burning pain in the gastric cavity which occurs now and then, exacerbation in the afternoon or in hunger, remission on food-entry, dry mouth with bitter taste, vexation and irritability, and poor appetite, which is called stomach-heat and yin-difficiency, also press-knead Yangling-quan (GB 34), Neiguan (PC 6) Weishu (BL 21) in addition.

5. Course of treatment: Once a day, 15 times as one course; with an interval of 5-7 days between two courses.

VII QIGONG THERAPEUTIC METHODS

1. Self-treatment by practising qigong
1) Basic Maneuvers
Choose Relaxation Qigong and Inner-Nourishing Qigong to practise.
2) Auxiliary maneuvers
(1) Stagnation of qi of the liver and stomach: It is advisable to practise the methods of rubbing the chest and training qi with the word"hu" as well as dredging the spleen and the stomach in Regulation-Spleen Qigong, rubbing the chest and training qi with the word "xu" as well as dredging the liver and conducting qi in Regulating-Liver Qigong.

(2) Deficiency of stomach-yin due to stomach-heat: It is advisable to practise the methods of taking yellow qi, dredging the spleen and the stomach in Regulating-Spleen Qigong as well as the "chui" -character in Six-character Formula.

(3) Weakness of both the spleen and stomach: It is advisable to practise Abdomen Qigong, Regulating-spleen Qigong and the methods of taking yellow

qi and taking red qi in Regulating-Heart Qigong.

2. External qi (Waiqi) therapy

1) Basic maneuvers

(1) Ask the patient to lie on his back, relax his whole body, get rid of stray thoughts, then conduct qi with mindwill to the stomach when exhaling.

(2) The therapist presses the patient's acupoint Lanmen (Ileocecal Junction, 1.5 cun above the navel) with the middle finger of the right hand, press the acupoint Jiuwei (below Xi-phoid, RN 15) with the middle finger of the left hand and use the regulating manipulation to open through the acupoint Lanmen (Ileocecal Junction, 1.5 cun above the navel).

(3) The therapist applies the flat-palm form, uses the vibrating and quivering manipulations to emit qi onto Zhong-wan (Middle Epigastrium, RN 12) and Liangmen (Beam Gate, ST 21) for 14 or 28 breaths respectively, then push the abdomen to the left and right, rub, knead and push the abdomen.

(4) Apply the flat-palm form, use the pushing, pulling, quivering and leading manipulations to emit qi onto Zhong-wan (Middle Epigastrium, RN 12), Liangmen (Beam Gate, ST 21) and Shanzhong (Middle Chest, RN 17), and conduct qi downward along the Ren Channel and the Stomach Channel.

(5) The patient lies pronely. Press and knead the patient's Pishu (Spleen shu, BL 20), Weishu (Stomach shu, BL 21) and the Urinary Bladder Channel on the Iumbodorsal region, from above to below.

2) Auxiliary Maneuvers

(1) Stagnation of qi of the liver and stomach: Apply the flat-palm form, use the pulling and leading manipulations to emit qi onto Ganshu(Liver Shu, BL 18), pull and conduct qi along the Gallbladder Channel and the Liver Channel down to the lower limbs so as to make qi balanced from left to right and from top to bottom.

(2) Deficiency of stomach-yin due to stomach-heat: Apply the flat-palm form, use the vibrating and quivering manipulations to emit qi onto Pishu(Spleen Shu, BL 20) and Shenshu (Kidney Shu, qi BL 23), and conduct qi downward along the Urinary Bladder Channel.

(3) Weakness of both the spleen and stomach: Apply the flat-palm form, use the pushing and pulling manipulations to emit qi onto the acupoints Qihai(Qi Sea, RN 6), Dantian(Elixir Field) and Guanyuan(Energy Pass, RN 4).

VIII MEDICATED DIET

1) Stomach-warming chicken (Nuan wei Ji)

INGREDIENTS

Rhizoma Zingiberis Recens	6g
Fructus Amoni	3g
Flos Caryophylli	3g
Rhizoma Alpiniae Officinarum	3g
Cortes Cinnamomi	3g
Pericarpium Citri Reticulatae	3g
Fructus Anisi Stellati	3g
Bulbus Allii Fistulisi	right amount
Soy asuce and table salt	right amount
Pepper powder	a little

PROCESS Skin the roaster, get rid of the entrails, wash it clean, cut in into pieces and put them in an earthenware pot with all the other ingredients but the pepper powder and a right amount of water; then stew it over slow fire, and when it is done, scatter the pepper powder on it.

DIRECTIONS The meat is for eating and the soup for drink. It is to be taken as much as one thinks it fit each time. It is used to treat stomachache of asthenia-cold type or stomach-cold type.

2) Gruel Activting qi and promoting digestion (Xingqi Jianwei zhou)

INGREDIENTS

Furctus Amoni	3g
Pericarpium Citri Reticulatae	6g
Fructus Aurantii	6g
Fructus Citri Sarcodactylis	6g
Semen Oryzae Sativae	100g

PROCESS Decoct the first four ingredients, sift the decoction from the dregs; then put the rice into the decoction with a right amount of water and make them into gruel.

DIRECTIONS To be taken twice each day for treatment of stomachache marked by the types of stagnation of qi.

3) Three-immortal gruel with additions (Jiawei sanxian zhou)

INGREDIENTS

Massa Fermentata Medicinalis	12g
Fructus Crataegi	12g
Fructus Hordei Germinatus Praeparatus	12g
Oryzae Germinatus Praeparatus	12g
Pericarpium Citri Reticulatae	6g
Semen Oryzae Sativae	100g

PROCESS Decoct the first five ingredients in water, remove the dregs from the decoction; then add in the rice and a right amount of water and cook them into gruel.

DIRECTIONS To be taken twice each day. It is applicable to stomachache of indigestion type.

4) Egg steamed with notoginseng and lotus root juice (Sanqi ouzhi Dun Ji-dan)

INGREDIENTS

Egg	1
Succus Rhizomatis Nelumbinis	30ml
Pulvis Radicis Notoginseng	3g

PROCESS First beat the egg in a bowl, put in the other two ingredients and mix them well; then steam it by putting the bowl in boiling water in a pot.

DIRECTIONS To be taken once or twice a day. Applicable to patients suffering from stomachache of blood stasis type.

5) Drink of fragrant solomonseal rhizome, dendrobium, black plam and hawthorn fruit (Yu shi mei zha yin)

INGREDIENTS

Rhizoma Polygonati	6g
Odorati	6g
Herba Dendrobii	6g
Fructus Crataegi	6g
Radix Paeoniea Alba	6g
Fructus Mume	3g
Radix Glycyrrhizae	3g

PROCESS Decoct in water all of the ingredients.

DIRECTIONS To be taken as a drink. It is applicable to stomachache marked by syndrome of deficiency of yin, and also good for atrophic gastritis marked by hypochlorhydria.

6) Pork stomach stewed with pepper and amomum fruit (Hujiao sharen Dun zhudu)

INGREDIENTS

Pork stomach	1
Fructus Piperis Nigri	6g
Fructus Amomi	6g
Rhizoma Zingiberis	6g
Pericarpium Citri Reticulatae	3g
Cortex Cinnamomi	3g
Bulbus Allii Fistulosi	right amount
Soy sauce and table salt	right amount

PROCESS First wash the pork stomach clean, place it kin an earthenware pot with a right amount of water, and add in all the ingredients; then stew it over slow fire until it is well-done.

DIRECTIONS To be taken as much as the patient thinks it fit. It is used to treat stomachache of stomach-cold type or asthcnia-cold type.

7) Gruel of galangal rhizome and cyperus tuber (Liang fu zhou)

INGREDIENTS

Rhizoma Alpiniae Officinarum	9g
Rhizoma Cyperi	9g
Semen Oryzae Satiuae	100g

PROCESS Decoct the first two ingredients in water, sift the decoction from the dregs; then add the rice and a right amount of water to the decoction and make them into gruel.

DIRECTIONS To be taken twice each day; it is applicable to patients suffering from stomachache of stomach-cold type or that accompanied with symptoms of stagnation of qi.

8) Drink of tangerine peel with additions (Fufang Jupi cha)

INGREDIENTS

Pericarpium Citri Reticulatae (which must be cut into threads)	6g

Fructus Citri Sarcodactylis (which must be cut into threads)　　6g

Flos Rosae Rugosae　　3g

PROCESS Infuse all the three ingredients in boiling water.

DIRECTIONS To be taken as a drink. Its indications are the same as those of Gruel Activationg Qi and Promotiong Digestion.

9) Cake for warming the middle-jiao and strengthening the stomach (wenzhong jianwei bing)

INGREDIENTS

Rhizoma Dioscoreae　　60g

Rhizoma Atractyloidis Macrocephalae　　60g

Poria　　60g

Rhizoma Zingiberis　　30g

Pericarpium Citri Reticulatae　　15g

Fructus Piperis Nigri　　3g

Flour　　1000g

PROCESS First grind together the first five ingredients into fine powder and mix them well with the pepper powder; Then mix the well-mixed powder with the flour and water into dough and make small cakes like biscuits; finally bake the small cakes in an oven.

DIRECTIONS This cake is applicable to those who suffer from stomachache of asthenia-cold type. It is to be taken at usual time as much as the patient thinks it fit and at any time he or she wishes.

Chapter Two
Gastroduodenal Ulcers

Gastroduodenal ulcers rank on the list of common and frequently occurring internal diseases and mostly affected among adolescent or middle-aged patients. Peptic ulcers are more frequently found in males than females. they are chronic in nature and often relapse. Clinically, their symptoms include periodic and rhythmic pain, accompanied by acid regurgitation, belching and vomiting etc. The ulcers can occur singularly or in multiple locations along the gastroduodenal tract. The coexistence of gastric and duodenal bulb ulcer is referred to as a complex ulcer. In severe cases, perforation, massive hemorrhage, pyloric stenosis and canceration may occur.

The incidence of duodenal ulcer has been declining at a rate of about 8% per yeat for the past decade. Although the average age at onset is 33, duodenal ulcer may occur at any time from infancy to the later years. It is 4 times as common in males as in females. Occurrence during pregnancy iis unusual.

Duodenal ulcer is 4 or 5 times as common as benign gastric ulcer. Morbidity due to peptic ulcer is a major bublic health problem.

About 95% of duodenal ulcers occur in the duodenal bulb or cap, i. e. the first 5cm of the duodenum. The remainders are between this area and the ampulla. Ulcers below the ampulla are rare. The ulceration varies from a few millimeter to 1-2cm in diameter and extends at least through the muscularis mucosae, often through to the serosa and into the pancreas. The margins are sharp, but the surrounding mucosa is often inflamed and edematous. The base consists of granulation tissue and fibrous tissue, representing healing and continuing digestion. In TCM, the disease is categorised as " epigastric pain ", " acid regugitation"or "distress in the stomach ".

I ETIOLOGY AND PATHOGENESIS

The digestive action of hydrochloric acid and pepsin on the mucosa causes ulcers in the upper gastrointestinal tract. Thus, these became known as "peptic ulcers ". Its pathogenic factors include deficiency and excessiveness, deficiency refers to the deficiency in the spleen and stomach, excessiveness refers to those pathogenic factors which irritate the stomach. the latter include catching cold, eating too much raw and cold food, or improper ingestion leading to food stagnancy, dyspesia and endogenous damp-heat, and blocked Qi stemming from liver dysfunction and affectiong stomach. This may turn into heat or leed to blood stasis.

II MAIN POINTS OF DIAGNOSIS

1. Symptoms: Cardinal symptom of the disease is chronic epigastralgia which is marked by dull pain or pinching pain. Sometimes it is manifested as distending pain or burning pain which often radiates to the lumbar region or the back. The pains are closely related to meals. The rule of attack kin gastric ulcer is food intake→pain→remission, while in duodenal ulcer the rule is pain→food intake→remission. The pain occurs periodically and is often induced by coldness, fatigue and improper food intake. The attack is frequently kin winter and spring.

Other symptoms include acid regurgiation, belching, nausea and vomiting. In a few cases, perforation or bleeding may be the first clinical findings.

2. Signs: In active ulcer, there is often tenderness in the middle and upper abdominal regions. Tendrness on the left side of upper gastric region is found in gastric ulcer, while in duodenal ulcer it is found on the right side, often localized in 3-4cm. Ulcer in the posterior wall may have pain hypersensitive area on the back at TII-12 level.

3. Laboratory examinations

(1) Fecal occult blood test (OB): OB positive reaction after 3-day vegetarian meals reveals that the active ulcer exists.

OB positive result may turn into negative if the patient is treated properly. Persistent positive reaction indicates cancerous change of ulcer or gastric carcinoma.

(2) X-ray barium examnation: It is of great value. Niche is often seen in gastric ulcer. Indirect signs such as irritation and disformity of duodenal bulbar region may occur in duodenal ulcer.

(3) Fiberscope examination: It is a main diagnostic method. Small and superficial ulcer can be seen directly. If fiberscopy is combined with biopsy, benign and cancerous changes can be differentiated. Gastric juice analysis is not used as a routine examination.

III DIFFERENTIATION AND
TREATMENT OF COMMON SYNDROMES

1. Insufficiency-cold type

Main symptoms and signs: Latent pain in the upper abdomen with predilection for heat, and intolerance of cold which aggravates the pain, sallow complexion, lassitude and weakness, or loose stool, pale tongue with thin whitish fur, deep, slow and weak pulse.

Therpaeutic principle: Warming and invigorating middle-jiao.

Recipe: Modified Decoction of Astragalus for Tonifying Middle-jiao.

Radix Astragali seu Hedysari	30g
Ramulus cinnamomi	9g
Radix Paeoniae Alba	18g
Os sepiella seu Sepiae	30g
Radix Angelicae Dahuricae	15g
Radix Glycyrrhizae Praeparate	15g

All the above drugs are to be decocted in water for oral administration.

2. Qi-stagnation type

Main symptoms and signs: Epigastric distension and pain, distension and fullness in the hypochondria, belching, acid regugitation, poor appetite, thin and whitish coating of the tongue, and taut pulse.

Therapeutic principle: Soothing the liver, regulating the circulation of qi and regulating the function of stomach to relieve pain.

Recipe: Modified Powder for Treating Cold Limbs in Combination with Sichuan Chinaberry Powder.

Radix Bupleuri	9g
Rhizoma Cyperi	12g
Radix Paeoniae Alba	9g
Frucuts Aurnntii	9g
Pericarpium Citri Reticulatae	9g
Fructus Meliae Toosendan	12g
Rhizoma Corydalis	12g
Radix Aucklandiae	9g

Caulis Perillae	12g
Concha Arcae	30g
Fructus Citri Sarcodactylis	9g
Radix glycyrrhizae Praeparata	6g

All the above drugs are to be decocted in water for oral administration.

3. Stagnated-heat type

Main symptoms and signs: Epigastric pain which is aggravated after food intake, burning sensation in the stomach, dry mouth with bitter taste, fondness of cold drink, constipation, deep-coloured urine, red tongue with yellow fur, taut and rapid pulse.

Therapeutic principle: Clearing away pathogenic heat and regulating the function of stomach.

Recipe: Modified Two Old Drugs Decoction in combination with Decoction for Eliminating Pathogenic Heat from th e Liver.

Rhizoma Coptidis	9g
Fructus Gardeniae	9g
Radix Scutellariae	9g
Rhizoma Anemarrhenae	10g
Radix Paeoniae Alba	10g
Pericarpium Citri Reticulatae	9g
Rhizoma Pinelliae	10g
Poria	10g
Fructus Citri Sarcodactylis	10g
Herba Dendrobii	10g
Radix Glycyrrhizae Praeparata	6g

All the above drug are to be decocted in water for oral administration.

If the case is complicated with insufficiency of the stomach-yin marked by latent pain in the epigastric region, dry mouth with reduced saliva, hot sensation in the palms and soles, red tongue with litttle fur or absence of fur and taut weak pulse, it is preferable to administer the Modified decoction of Glehnia and Ophiopogon instead. Its compositions are: glehnia root (Radix Glehniae) 10g, ophiopogon root (Radix Ophiopogonis) 10g, fragrant solomonseal rhizome (Rhizoma Polygonati Odorati)10g, white hyaciath bean (Semen Dolichoris Album) 10g, finger citron (Fructus Citri Sarcodactylis)10g, dendrobium (Herba Dendrobii)

10g, prepared licorice root (Radix Glycyrrhizae Praeparata)6g. All the drugs in the above recipe are to be decocted in water for oral administration.

If the case is manifested as severe symptom of blood stasis such as epigastric stabbing pain, or fixed pain just like knifecutting, dark purple tongue or with ecchymoses, taut or unsmooth pulse, the modified Red Sage Drink in combination with Wonderfgul Powder for Reliving Blood Stagnation is preferable: red sage root (Radix Salviae Miltiorrhizae)20g, amomum fruit (Fructus Amomi) 10g, cat-tail pollen(Pollen Typhae) 10g, trogopterus dung (Faeces Trogopterorum) 10g, sichuan chinaberry (Fructus Meliae Toosendan) 12g, corydalis tuber(Rhizoma Corydalis) 12g, Chinese angelica root (Radix Angelicae Sinensis) 12g, red peony root (Radix Paeoniae Rubra) 10g, prepared licorice root (Radix glycyrrhizae Praeparate)6g. All the above drugs are to be decocted in water for oral administration. For the case with hematemesis and tarry stools, 6 grams of powder of hyacinth bletilla (Radix Bletillae) and 3 grams of powder of notoginseng (Radix Notoginseng) should be added (administered orally after being mixed with the finished decoction). The above drugs except powder of notoginseng are to be decocted in water for oral administration.

4. Intense fire in the gallbladder and stomach

Main symptoms and signs: Urgent stomachache with burning sensation, acid regurgitation, feeling of distress in the stomach, eating much food but still easily getting hungry, preference for cold drinks, nausea, thirst and bitter taste in the mouth, red tongue with yellow coating, rapid and taut pulse.

Recipe:

Radix Thalictrum	1g
Fructus Evodiae	5g
Pericarpium Citri Reticulatea	5g
Rhizoma Pinelliae	10g
Poria	10g
Fructus Aurantii Immaturus	10g
Caulis Bambusae in Taenis	10g
Fructus Gardeniae	10g
Concha Arcae	10g
Os Sepiae	10g
Frictus Trichosanthis	10g

All above drugs were decocted in water for oral use. One dese of the Recipe wao given daily for two times of taking.

All cases of the mentioned above-types should add some patent medicines such as Granule for Qi-stagnancy and Stomachache, Pills for Nourishing Spleen with Radix Ginseng, "Zuo Jin"Pills, etc.

68 cases were treated with the above method. After 2-4 years, follow up and only in 9 cases did the symptoms recur. The shortest recurrent time was 3 months, the longest recurrent time was 3 and a half years. The total recurrent rate was only 12.9%. Cancer occurred in no cases.

5. Attack of stagnated liver qi on the stomach

Main symptoms and signs: Distending pain in the opigastric region, acid regurgitation and belching, aggravated by anxiety and mental depression, thin, white tongue coating and taut pulse.

If stagnated liver qi lasts for a long time, it may turn into heat, manifested as thirst, reddened tongue with yellow coating and rapid and taut pulse.

Stagnated liver qi may also cause blood stasis, which is characterized by localized stabbing pain aggravated by pressure, dark purple tongue or with petechiae, thin, white tongur coating and hesitant pulse.

Principle of treatment: Disperse stagnated liver qi and harmonize the stomach.

Recipe: Chaihu shugan San (Bupleurum Powder for soothing the Liver); if the syndrome is complicated by blood stasis, Rhizoma Corydalis, Radix Salviae Miltiorrhizae and Faeces Trogopterorum may be added to promote blood circulation and eliminate blood stasis.

6. Accumalation of phlegm-damp in the middle-jiao

Main symptoms and signs: Epigastric pain occurring after meals, thirst without preference for drink, poor appetite, white and greasy tongue coating and smooth pulse. Thesr symptoms indicate a phlegm-damp syndrome of the cold type. If the tongue becomes red with a yellow and greasy coating and the patient experiences thirst, concentrated urine and constipation, the phlegm-damp syndrome has turned into damp-heat. Principle of treatment: Strengthen the spleen and eliminate phlegm-damp.

Recipe: Erchen Decoction (Decotion of Two Old Drugs) and Liang Fu Wan (Galangal and Cyperus Pill); Poria and Radix glycyrrhizae Praeparata strengthen the spleen and dispel damp; Rhizoma Pinelliae Praeparata is used with Poria and Radix Glycyrrhizae to strengthen the effect of dispelling phlegm-damp; Pericarpium Citri Reticulatae, Rhizoma Cyperi and Rhizoma Alpiniae regulate qi and relieve pain; if the phlegm-damp has turned into phlegm-heat, it should be treated with Banxia Xiexin Tang (Pinellia Decoction for Purging Stomach Fire); in this formula, Rhizoma Coptidis and Radix Scutellariae dispel internal heat, Rhizoma Zingiberis and Rhizoma Pinelliae dispel phlegm and Rdix Ginseng, Radix Glycyrrhizae Praeparata and Fructus Ziziphi Jujubae strengthen the spleen and harmonize the stomach.

IV   LOCAL TDREATMENT

Ma Liansheng et al combined local treatment with orally administered Chinese herbs to treat the disease.

Method: The ulcerative surface was debrided under and endoscope. 8 ml (containing 40 mg) of anisodamini hydrobromidum and 4 ml (containing 6g) of injectio Radix Salviae Milttiorrhizae were injected at the border between the ulcer's bottom and the ulcer's edge through an injection needle of the endoscope. 4-5 points were injected each time at the place between mucous membrane and the muscular layer. Finally 20 ml of 50% mixed solution (prepared with Rhizoma Bletillae, Radix Notoginseng etc) were directly injected on the ulcerative surface until the surface was completely covered. One time of treatment was given every 7 days. The treatment was usually repeated 2-3 times when required. After the operation, 45 g of the "chuan Jia Wei Tan " infusion (containing Squama Manitis 6g, Radix Astrogali seu Hedysari12g, Radix Notoginseng 5 g, Rhizoma coptidis 5g, Herba Asari 3 g and Rhizoma Bletillae 10g) was taken twice daily in the morning and evening. 4 weeks were set as a course of treatment.

90 cases of gastric ulcer were treated. Ulcers in 86 cases were healed (95. 6%). Among 170 cases of duodenal ulcer, ulcers in 150 cases were healed (88. 2%). The relief rates of main symptoms were 70% and 97% in the first week and second week of the treatment respectively; the disappearance rates of pyloric spirillium were 71. 2% (GU) and 78. 3% (PU) respectively.

V ACUPUNCTURE AND MOXIBUSTION

1. Body acupunture therapy:

1) Main Points: Weishu(BL 21), Ganshu(BL 18), Zhongwan(RN 12), Zusanli(ST 36),

Supplementary points: Liangmen(ST 21), Neiguan(PC 6), Sanyinjiao(SP 6).

Method: 2 or 3 of each of the main and auxiliary points are punctured with either moderate or strong stimulation. The needles are retained for 20 minutes and the therapy is given once daily.

2) Main points: Zhongwan (RN12) , Neiguan (PC6), and Zusanli (ST36).

Supplementary points: Add Qimen (LR14) and Yanglingquan (GB34) for the liver qi attacking the stomach; add Pishu (BL20), Weishu (BL21) and Zhangmen(LR13) for the deficiency and cold of the spleen and stomach.

Method: the reducing method is used for the excessive type; the reinforcing method for the deficient type. the points are punctured with the filiform needles.

2. Ear acupuncture therapy

1) Points: Stomach pt, Sympathetic Nerve pt, Subcortex pt and Duodemum pt.

Method: Select 2 or 3 of the abvoe points for each treatment. The needles are retained for 15 to 30 minutes. A course includes ten treatments and between courses the treatment is ceased for 2 or 3 days.

2) Prescribed Points: Stomach, Liver, Infraantihelix Crus End, Ear-shenmen, and Brain.

Method: Select 2 or 3 points for each treatment; twist the needles with strong stimulation; retain the needles for 20 to 30 minutes.

3. Electro-acupuncture

Fan Wansheng applied the method to treat perforation of acute peptic ulcer.

Points selected:

Main points: Zhongwan(RN 12).

Complementary points: Zusanli (ST 36) and Hegu (LI 4).

Method: Strong stimulation of electro-acupuncture was given for half an hour each time. An interval of 15 minutes was necessary between the two times fo stimulation. 8 hours' successive stimulation followed, when patient's pain was relieved, abdominal muscle relaxed, and the tenderness and rebound tenderness lessened, the stimulation was suspended. During the treatment of electroacupuncture, patients were given gastroenteric decompression and sufficient antibiotics. 48 hours later, Drastic Purgative Decoction might be taken. During the treatment, patients were instructed to lie in semisupination to prevent abscess under the diaphagm.

28 cases were treated with the method. 24 cases were cured. 4 cases were transfered to surgery to accept operation during the treatment process.

4. Point injection

Points selected:

Main points: Zusanli (ST 36), Zhongwan (RN 12), Weicang (BL 50) (right), Pishu (BL 20) (right).

Complementary points: for abdominal distension, Yanglingquan (GB 34) was added; for nausea and vomiting, Jianjing (GB 21) and Neiguan (PC 6) were added.

Method: 5 ml syringe was used to draw 2 ml (o. 2 g) of injection cimetidine which was diluted to 5 ml with normal saline. No. 4 needle was used to insert into the points. After patients felt needling sensation of soreness, numbness and distension, the drug solution was slowly injected into the points About 1ml of it was given for each point. 3-4 points were selected each time. One time of the treatment was done daily. 14 times of the injection were set as a course of treatment.

After 2 courses of treatment, 40 cases out of 50 cases were cured (80%); 6 cases gained obvious effect (12%); 2 cases somewhat improved(4%).

5. Thread embedding therapy in points

1) Main points: Penetrating Shangwan (RN 13) from Zhougwan (RN 12), Penetrating Pishu (BL 20) from Weishu (BL 12), Zusanli (ST 36).

Supplementary points: For cases with periodic epigastric pain accompanied by abdominal distension, nausea, vomiting, belching and acid regurgitation, Liangqiu (ST 34) was added; for cases with radiating, pain to the hypochondria, belching, acid regurgitation, taut and thin pulse, Taichong (LR 3) and Qimen (LR 14) were added; for cases with accumulation of fluid in the stomach, deep and taut pulse, Sanjiaoshu (BL 22) was added; for cases with epigastric pain which could be relieved by applying pressur, regurgitation of thin fluid, deep, slow, thin and weak pulse, Mingmen (DU 4) was added; for cases with foul brerth, constipation, pain in the epigastrium which was hard while being pressed, Neiting (ST 44) and Fenglong (ST 40) were added; for cases with fixed pain, hemafecia, tongue with spots of stagnant blood at its edges, Ganshu (BL 18) and Geshu (BL 17) were added; for cases with gastroptosis, Weishang (Extra 14), Baihui (DU 20), Qihai (RN 6) and Shenshu (BL 23) were added; for cases with severe vomiting, Neiguan (PC 6) was added.

Method: Only the main points were selected in the first group (1078 cases). Routine No. O catgut suture was embedded in these points for one time in a month. The total point-embeding times were uncertain. In the second group (186 cases); not only were the main points selected, but alsothe coplementary were added, on the basis of symjptom-sign differentiation. Routine No. O catgut suture was embeded in these points for one time a month. A total of 3-6 times of embedding was necessary. In the third group (100 cases), the selection of points was the same as that of the scond group. Routine No. O catgut suture was embeded in these points for one time a month for a total of 6 times, and in the mean time, powder of Peptic Ulcer was taken 3 times an day at 6 g each time over a succession of 2 weeks.

In the first group, 28.7% of the cases were cured; 56.4% of the cases gained obvious effect; and the total effective rate was 85.1%. In the second group, 46.2% of the xases were cured, 38.2% of the cases gained obvious effect, and the total effective rate was 84.4%; in the third group, 83% of the cases were cured, 4% of the cases gained obvious effect, and the total effective rate was 87%.

2) Points selected: Penetrating Shangwan (RN 13) from Zhongwan (RN 12), penetrating the bilateral Pishu (BL 20) from the bilateral Weishu (BL 21).

Method: After local sterilization, 1-2 ml of 0.25-0.5% procaine hydrochloride was injected into each point for local anaesthesia. No 0-1 sterile chromicized catgut suture was used and connected to a three-edged bent needle of stainless steel. The doctor pinched up the skin around the point with hios left hand and used a needle-holder to penetrate the bottom of the two points at the originally selected place with his right hand. The free side of the suture was drawn to hypoderm of the needle insertion site. the other side of the suture was cut against skin and then massaged to make the suture side wijthdraw under the skin. The treatment was given once in a month.

218 cases were treated, 150 cases were cured (68. 8%). 54 cases gained some effect (24. 3%). the total effective rate was 93. 6%.

6. Cupping therapy

Cupping is applied with erther large or medium-sized cups mainly on the upper abdomen, or the Back-shu points for 10 to 15 minutes.

VI MASSAGE

Push to and fro from Zhongwan (RN 12) upward to Shangwan (RN 13) and to the xiphoid process with the soft and light one-finger push method for 5 to 10 minutes; with Zhongwan (RN 12) as the centre, rub clockwise and counterclockwise for 200 to 300 times respectively. Then vibrate the upper abdomen for 3 to 5 minutes; press and knead Zusanli (ST 36), Ganshu (BL 18), Danshu (BL19), Qimen (LR 14), Zhangmen (LR 13), Neiguan (PC 6), Dachangshu (BL 25), and Yanglingquan (GB 34)for 5 minutes respectively; push or press and knead Pishu (BL 20), Weishu (BL 21) or Ashi points on the back for 2 to 3 minutes respectively with the one-finger push method.

VII QIGONG

1. Assume the standing or sitting posture. Relax the whole body; breathe naturally and get rid of distracting thoughts. First knock the teeth for 36 times; stir the saliva inside the mouth with the tongue; swallow the saliva in 3 parts and send it with the mind to the location of Zhongwan (RN 12) above the naval. Then imagine a yellow qi; breathe it in and fill the whole mouth with it; when exhaling, send it slowly to the location of Zhongwan (RN 12) and further to the four limbs, skin and hair. Do it this way for 5 to 10 times.

2. Assume the sitting or standing posture. Gently place the right palm flat on the location of Zhongwan (RN 12) on the upper abdomen and exhale slowly.

When exhaling, rub the right palm clock-wise; meanwhile utter "Hu". Do for 10 or 20 breaths.

3. Assume the standing or sitting posture. Place both palms flat on both sides of the chest and inhale slowly. When exhaling, read "xu"; meanwhile gently rub both costal regions in circular motion with both palms. Do for 10 or 20 breaths.

VIII   MEDICATED DIET

1. Stew a pig's stomach after it has been washed clean with 6g of black pepper, 9g of amomum fruit, 6g of dried ginger, 6g of tangerine peel, 3g of cassia bark and a right amount of green Chinese onion, soy sauce and salt in an earthware pot with a right amount of water over slow fire until it is well done. Take it in proper proportion. It is used to treat the stomachache of the deficient-cold type.

2. Infuse 9g of shredded tangerine peel and 6g of finger citron, together with 3g of dried rose, in boiling water to drink as tea. It is suitable to the stomachache of yin deficiency.

3. Decoct 9g of fragrant solomonseal rhizome, 6g of dendrobium, 6g of hawthorn fruit, 6g white peony root, 6g of black plum, and 3g of licorice root in water to drink as tea. It is applicable to the stomachache of yin deficiency.

IX   TREATMENT OF COMPLICATIONS

1. Hemorrhage

Acute bleeding is serious complication of peptic ulcers. Here again, traditional Chinese methods combined with Western medical techniques resulted in benefical effects.

Traditional Chinese medicine holds that acute hemorrhage in peptic ulcer is caused by: a) accummulation of heat in the stomach brought on by taking too much heat-propertied food or an attack of pathogenic heat damaging the collaterals of the stomach; b) heat transformed from stagnated liver qi attacking the stomach; and c) deficiency of spleen qi failing to keep the blood flowing within the vessels.

Differential diagnosis of syndromes and treatment:

1) Bbleeding dur to accummulation of heat in the stomach

Main symptoms and signs: Distending pain over the epigastrium and abdomen, hematemesis, thirst with preference for cold dring, scanty urine, constipation, reddened tongue with yellow coating and rapid pulse.

Principle of treatment: Cleat away heat from the stomach, remove blood stasis and arrest bleeding.

Recipe: Qingwei San (Powder for Clearing Stomach Fire) plus Shihui San (Powder of Ashes of Ten Drugs) with modifications.

2) Bleeding due to the liver heat attacking the stomach

Main symptoms and signs: Nausea, hematemesis, bitter taste in the mouth, hypochondriac distending pain, irritability, excitabillity, reddened tongue and taut pulse.

Principle of treatment: clear away pathogenic heat from the liver and stomach and stop bleeding by cooling the blood.

Recipe: Longdan Xiegan Tang (Decoction of Gentian for Purging Liver Fire) plus Cortex Moutan Radicis, Fructus Gardeniae and Radix Scutellariae.

3) Bleeding due to deficiency of spleen and stomach qi

Main symptoms and signs: Pallid complxion, lassitude and weakness, shortness of breath, abdominal distension, nausea, hematemesis, pale tongue and small, deep pulse.

Principle of treatment: Resplenish qi to arrest bleeding.

Recipe: Guipi Tang (Docoction for Invigorating the Spleen and Nourishing the Heart) with modifications.

In serious cases, the following emergency treatments are recommended in addition to blood transfusions.

1) Rhizoma Bletillae Powder (10g) plus White Drug Powder (2g): Make into a paste with 150 ml warm boiled water; 15 ml taken orally every 2 hours on the first day; if the blecding stops, the dosage may be reduced to 15 ml 4 times a day fro 3 days.

2) Rhubarb Powder: 3 g 3 times a day taken orally. an alcoholic extract of rhubarb (AER) in treating 182 cases of upper gastrointestinal hemorrhage. (AER) achieved a total effective rate of 96. 1 percent with hemostasis occurring

in two-to-eight days. The common causes of bleeding were peptic ulcer, gastritis and neoplasm of the stomach, the mechanisms of AER responsible for hemostasis include contraction of the local blood vessels, reduction in permeability and motility of the small intestine and inhibition of pepsin activity. Elevation of the plasma osmotic pressure may also contribute to hemostasis. Pharmacological studies indicate that rhubarb has two active hemostatic components: d-catechin and gallic acid.

3) Alumen: 35 cases of gastric bleeding treated with a 6 percent Alumen Solution which was directly injected to the bleeding sites using gastroscopy. Hemostasis occurred within one minute in 34 cases, and within two minutes in one case. This solution can also be used orally for treating gastric bleeding.

4) Folium Sennae: The effect of Folium Sennae on acute gastroduodenal hemorrhage in 340 cases. A powder of Folium Sennae was administered orally at a dose of 1 g 3 times a day. After the treatment, hemostasis occurred in 320 cases (94. 1 percent), and the average hemostatic time was 2. 68±0. 12 days, as judged by the absence of occult blood in the feces. A control group of 100 patients reccived Cimetidin. Their hemostatic rate was 90 percent, and the average hemostatic time was 4. 5±0. 16 days. Experiments showed that coaglation time, thromboplastin time and clot retraction time were remarkably shortened after administering Folium Sennae.

2. Perforation

Western physicians typically indicate surgery in peptic ulcer patients with perforation, hemorrhage or obstruction. In the past 30 years, however, Chinese physicians have studied the effects of combined traditional Chinese and western medical treatment of perforated peptic ulcers. this type of treatment is indicated in patients under 60 years old who are in good general condition, have normal blood pressure, pulse and respiration, show no obvious abnormalities of the heart, lungs, liver and kidneys, have had a short course of peptic uler and an absence of shifting dullness in the abdomen and whose body temperature is less than 39 ℃. The therapeutic regimen consists of three stages.

First stage: The patient should be in a semi-reclining position; no food intake is allowed. The main treatment includes gastrointestinal decompression, intravenous infusion with antibiotics and electrically stimulated acupuncture. The principal acupoints are Zusanli (ST 36), zhongwan(RN 16), Tianshu(ST 25) and Liangmen (ST 21). The needles should be retained for 12-24 hours, with electric stimulation every two hours for 30 minutes each time. The patient should be closely observed for 12-24 hours. If the patient's condition improves, the treatment can be continued; otherwise, surgical intervention should be given at once. Experimental studies revealed the multiple effects of acupuncture therapy in this stage: to inhibit the secretion of gastric fluid, acid and pepsin; to promote the restoration of peristalsis and the opening of the pylorus to evacuate the gastric content; and to increase the phagocytic function.

Second stage: Clearing away heat and counteracting toxicity are the main principles of treatment in this stage. Use Da Chaihu Tang (Major Bupleurum Decoction) with modifications for 5-7 days. When the patient recovers his appetite, his body temperature will return to normal, his symptoms will basically disappear and he is ready for the third stage of treatment.

Studies have shown that Major Bupleurum Decoction is anti-inflammator and antibiotic, and restores gastrointestinal functions and promotes absorption of abdominal exudate.

Third stage (convalescence): Here treatment is aimed at curing the peptic ulcer. In cases of excess-heat type, the treatment involves clearing heat and purging fire, using Banxia Xiexin Tang (Pinellia Decoction for Purging Stomach Fire) with modifications. In cases of deficiency-cold type, therapy involves replenishing qi and warming middle-jiao, using Liu Junzi Tang (Decoction of Six Noble Ingredients) or Lizhong Tang (Decoction for Regulating Middle-jiao) with modifications.

In 5,920 cases of ulcerative perforation treated with the combined therapy, the cure rate was 92. 4 percent, the mortality rate 0. 8 percent. Physicians followed 652 of these cases for five years. Of them, 83. 4 percent experienced satisfactory results, while only 11. 5 percent needed a gastrectomy.

Chapter Three
Viral Hepatitis

Viral hepatitis, is caused by hepatitis viruses. People are susceptible to the disease. Clinically, the major symptoms are poor appetite, hepatalgia and fatigur. Fever and jaundice may occur. Liver function test shows various degrees of hepatic damage. This refers to inflammation of the liver with little or no fibrosis and little or no nodular regeneration. There may be minor distortion of lobular architecture.

In TCM, this disease belongs to the categories of "huang dan"(jaundice), "gan yu"(stagnation of liver-qi), "xie tong"(hypochondriac pain) and "zheng ji"(mass in the abdomen).

I THREE MAJOR GROUPS OF ACUTE VIRAL HEPATITIS

1) Hepatitis A (infectious hepatitis IH, short incubation hepatitis).

2) Hepatitis B (serum hepatitis SH, long incubation hepatitis).

3) Non-A, non-B hepatitis which clinically resembles hepatitis B.

Australia antigen consists of morphologically identifiable particles. This antigen is present during acute episodes of hepatitis B and (usually) disappears as the hepatitis resolves.

1. Hepatitis A

The disease is caused by and enterovirus (hepatitis A antigen) which is excreted in the stools towards the end of the incubation period and disappears as the illness develops. antibody appears at the onset of the illness and a rising titre indicates recent infection. The disease is endemic but small epidemics may occur in schoold or institutions. spread is usually via the faecaloral route. It may be spread by food products such as shellfish. The young (5-14 years) are chiefly involved.

Clinical symptoms and signs:

After a variable incubation period of 2-6 weeks there is a gradual onset of an influenza-like illness with fever, malaise, anorexia, nausea, vomiting and upper abdominal discomfort associated with tender enlargement of the liver and, less commonly, the spleen. After 3-4 days the urine becomes characteristically dark and the stools pale-evidence of cholestasis. Symptoms usually become less severe as jaundice appears although pruritus may develop. Jaundice and symptoms tend to improve after 1-2 weeks and recovery is usually complete, although mild symptoms may continue for up to 3-4 months in a few patients. Recurrent hepatitis is extremely rare and immunity probably lifelong.

Management

If hospitalised the patient should be isolated. The true period of infectivity is unknown but is probably about 1-2 weeks after the appearance of jaundice. Symptomatic treatment only is required in the active disease state. Most physicians would restrict activity until jaundice has disappeared and allow moderate exertion whilst the serum transaminase levels remain elevated. No food restriction is necessary but alcohol should be avoided for at least 1 year. Liver function tests usually return completely to normal in 1-3 months.

Recovery is the rule in virtually every case. Occasionally jaundice may be prolonged by in tra-hepatic cholestasis, and corticosteroids can be used to reduce the jaundice rapidly. Particularly if it is associated with pruritus. In a small number of patients (5-10%) a mild relapse occurs, sometimes after the jaundice has disappeared. Acute massive necrosis is an extremely rare complication but invariably fatal.

Prophylaxis

Immune γ-globulin (500-750 mg in adults) protects contacts of infectious hepatitis. It is given to travellers entering endemic areas but the period of effectiveness remains uncertainprobably about 3-4 months.

2. Hepatitis B

This is spread by infected blood or serum and also occurs in salive, semen and vaginal secretions. It is most frequently seen in heroin addicts who use contaminated syringes and needles, and less commonly in patients and staffs in renal dialysis units and those attending centres for tattooing or acupuncture. Blood transfusion units now screen all donor blood for the presence of hepatitis B virus. Recent work has shown that the disease can also be transmitted by ingestion, although this must be very uncommon.

Clinical symptoms and signs

After a long incubation period of 6 weeks to 6 months, there is a gradual onset of lethargy, anorexia, abdominal discomfort, jaundice, and hepatomegaly. Arthralgia and skin rashes are common.

Diagnosis

Hepatitis B has a surface antigen (HBsAg) and a core antigen (HBcAg). The former appears in the blood about 6 weeks after infection, just before jaundice appears, and has usually gone by 3 months. In about 5% it persists beyond 6 months (carrier status) and the patient can transmit the disease even though well. The prevalance of carrier status varies from 1 to 2 per 1000 in UK and USA to 10-15% in parts of Africa and the Far East. The 'e' antigen found only in the presence of HBsAg, appears in the blood at the same time as the surface antigen and indicates high infectivity. Surface antibody (anti-HBs) appears in the blood about 3 months after infection and remains conferring immunity in 80-90% of cases.

Management and prognosis

While in hospital patients should be isolated, barrier nursed, and all excretion products disinfected. Blood samples should be taken wearing gloves, transported in plastic bags and the laboratory informed of the suspected diagnosis.

In uncomplicated cases treatment is symptomatic as for infectious hepatitis. Complications include chronic hepatitis, acute necrosis and liver failure which are more common following serum hepatitis than following infectious hapatitis. Carriers have a high incidence of hapatoma in the developing world.

Gamma globulin from blood containing specific hepatitis B antibodies can be given to those without the antibody who have been exposed to infection preferably within a few days.

3. Non-A non-B hepatitis

The infective agents transmit infection and confer specific immunity. It may clinically resemble infectious mononucleosis or cytomegalovirus infection and these must be excluded. A mild chronic hepatitis is relatively common(25%).

II ETIOLOGY AND PATHOGENESIS

Epidemi pathogens or pathogenic demp-heat accumulated in the interior of the body cause viral hepatitis.

1. Epidemic pathogens infect the liver and gallbladder, which results in heat or damp-heat that affects the smooth flow of liver qi and secretion of bile and leads to jaundice, anorexia and malaise.

2. Improper diet or abnormal weather causes dysfunction of the spleen in transportation and transformation, leading to retention of damp-heat in the spleen and gallbladder.

3. Exuberant pathogenic damp-heat accumulated in the interior of the body for a long time impairs vital essence; as a result, deficiency of yin, yang, qi or blood syndromes may occur. In serious cases, epidemic pathogens or damp-heat may invade the pericardium and cause coma or other central nervous symptoms.

III MAIN POINTS OF DIAGNOSIS

1. Epidemiologic information

The epidemic condition and a history of close contact with a hepatitis patient, or a history of blood transfusion, or receiving blood preparations or immunization injections should be noticed.

2. Clinical features

(1) The onset of the disease is insidious and slow. The patients often complain of fatigue and anorexia. Some have jaundice, but most of of them belong to the typs of non-icteric or mild hepatitis. Only ten percent of the patients have typical manifestations or jaundice.

(2) Patients with hepatitis A often manifest pyrexia, shorter course and rapid recovery; patients with hepatitis B usually have a chronic course and remain HB virus carriers for a long time. A few of them may progress to cirrhosis. The severity of the clinical features of Non-A Non-B hepatitis is between those of hepatitis A and hepatitis B. And its incubation period can be long or short.

3. Physical signs

The liver becomes enlarged, and tender on palpation and is painful on percussion. There is a mild change of liver texture. A small percentage of cases have splenomegaly. In the patients with icterohepatitis, jaundice may be found in the skin and sclera. Hepatic face, vascular spiders and liver palms may be present in chronic active hepatitis. A few patients suffering from fulminant hepatitis may have skin petechiae, epistaxis and ascites, or even hepatic coma, indicating poor prognosis.

4. Laboratory examination

(1) Liver function: In patients with acute hepatitis, the SGPT is marked elevated up to several hundreds units, even more than one thousand units. In icterohepatitis, the icterus index and the one-minute bilirubin fixed quantity are increased. In severe and chronic active hepatitis, metabolism of protein is disturbed resulting in the change of ratio of serum albumin to globulin. The albumin level lowered but the globulin level elevated, even the ratio may be inverted. Signs of clotting disorder may be present.

(2) The detection of specific antigens and antibodies: It is available to detect the HAAg in filtrate of stools and the antiHAV of the IgG and IgM class in the serum in the diagnosis of hepatitis A. Three antigen and antibody systems, that is HBsAg, HBcAg and HBeAg with their antibodies, can be detected, which is valuable in the diagnosis and in predicting tyhe severity, infectivity and prognosis of the hepatitis B. Non-A Non-B hepatitis can only be diagnosed by using the exclusive method.

(3) In chronic active hepatitis, tests for cellular immunity, humoral immunity and autoimmunity may be performed to evaluate the host immune mechanisms and severity of the disease so as to give a relevant treatment. Liver biopsy is only indicated for those whose cases defy diagnosis through clinical and laboratory examination.

IV DIFFERENTIATION AND
TREATMENT OF COMMON SYNDROMES

1. Icterohepatitis

(1) Yang Jaundice (Acute Icterohepatitis)

Main symptoms and signs: Bright yellow coloration of the skin and sclera, fever, thirst, feeling of fullness and distension in the epigastrium, anorexia, fatigue, hypochondriac distension and pain, restlessness, nausea, scanty dark urine, dry stools, red tongue with yellow and greasy fur, taut and rapid pulse.

Therapeutic principle: Removing pathogenic heat and dampness.

Recipe: Oriental Wormwood Decoction with additional ingredients.

Herba Artemisiae Capillaris	30g
Fructus Gardeniae	10g
Radix et Rhizoma Rhei (decocted later)	6g
Cortex Phellodendri	10g
Flos Lonicerae	30g
Fructus Forsythiae	15g
Radix Isatidis	30g
Rhizoma Imperatae	30g

All the above drugs are to be decocted in water for oral administration.

Some other drugs are often employed for certain symptoms. In case of exhibiting more symptoms and signs of pathogenic heat, 30 grams of isatis leaf (Folium Isatidis) and 30 grams of dandelion (Herba Taraxaci) should be added. And in case of exhibiting more symptoms and signs of pathogenic damp, 10 grams of atractylodes rhizome (Rhizoma Atractylodis), 10 grams of magnolia bark (Cortex Magnoliae Officinalis) and 10 grams of alismatis rhizome (Rhizoma Alismatis) may be added. Nausea and vomiting can be treated with the addition of pinellia tuber (Rhizoma Pinelliae) 10g and bamboo shavings (Caulis Bambusae in Taeniam) 10g. while abdominal distension and anorexia can be treated with the addition of same dosage of 10 grams of parched hawthorn fruit (Fructus Crataegi) parched malt (Fructus Hordei Germinatus) and parched medicated leaven (Massa Fermentata Medicinalis). To treat the cutaneous pruritus, 15 grams of dittany bark (Cortex Dictamni Radicis) and 15 grams of broom cypress fruit (fructus Kochiae) are included.

(2) Yin Jaundice (Chronic icterohepatitis)

Main symptoms and signs: Dark yellow coloration of the skin and sclera just like smoky colour, poor appetite, feeling of distension in the abdomen, loose stools, general debility, tastelessness in the mouth, whitish thick and greasy fur of the tongue, deep thready and weak pulse.

Therapeutic principle: Activating the function of the spleen, inducing diuresis and warming yang.

Redipe: Modified Decoction of Oriental Wormwood and Bighead Atractylodes and Prepared Aconite.

Herba Artemisiae Capillaris	30g
Rhizoma Atractylodis Macrocephalae	12g
Radix Codonopsis Pilosulae	12g
Poria	15g
Semen Coicis	30g
Radix Aconite Praeparata	6g
Pericarpium Citri Reticulatae	10g
Fructus Crataegi	10g
Fructus Hordei Germinatus	10g
Massa Fermentata Medicinalis	10g

All the above drugs are to be decocted in water for oral administration.

Apart from the ingredients in the above recipe, 10 grams of dried ginger (rhizoma Zingiberis) should be prescribed for those who complain of aversion to cold and cold limbs; 15 grams of fresh-water turtle shell (Carapax Trionycis) and 15 grams of red sage root (Radix Salviae Miltiorrhizae) for those with hepatosplenomegaly; and 15 grams of shell of areca nut (Pericarpium Arecae) and 15 grams of plantain seed (Semen Plantaginis, wrapped in a piece of cloth during decocting) for those with ascites.

2. Anicteric Hepatitis

(1) Dampness and heat in the liver and gallbladder

Main symptoms and signs: Chest stuffiness, dysphoria with feverish sensation, pain in the hypochondrium, abdominal distension, lassirude and weakness, anorexia with aversion to greasy food, bitter taste and dry mouth, scanty dark urine, dry stools, reddened tongue with yellow and gerasy fur, taut and rapid or smooth and rapid pulse.

Therapeutic principle: Removing pathogenic heat and dampness.

Recipe: Modified prescriptions of Oriental Wormwood Decoction combined with Decoction of Gentian for Purging Liver-fire.

Herba Artemisiae Capillaris	30g
Fructus Gardeniae	10g
Radix Scutellariae	10g

Radix Gentianae	10g
Radix Isatidis	30g
Herba Patriniae	30g
Radis Curcumae	12g
Semen Plantaginis	10g
(wrapped in a piece of cloth during decocting)	
Radix Salviae Miltiorrhizae	12g
Poria	10g
Cortex Magnoliae officinalis	10g

All the above drugs are to be decocted in water for oral administration.

In addition, 12 grams of Sichuan chinaberry (Fructus Meliae Toosendan) and 10 grams of corydalis tuber (Rhizoma Corydalis) are added for treating cases with prominent pain in the hypochondrium; 10 grams of amomum fruit (Fructus Amomi) and 10 grams of bitter orange (Fructus Aurantii) are added for cases with obvious epigastric distension and stuffiness; 15 grams of hawthorn fruit (Fructus Crataegi) and 10 grams of membrane of chicken's gizzard skin (Endothelium Corneum Gigeriae Calli) added for cases with poor appetite.

(2) Stagnation of the liver-qi with deficiency of the spleen

Main symptoms and signs: Dull pain in the right-sided hypochondrium, general debility, anorexia, loose stools, thin and whitish fur of the tongue, deep and taut pulse.

Therapeutic principle: Relieving the depressed liver-qi and reinforcing the function of the spleen.

Recipe: Modified Ease Powder.

Radix Bupleuri	10g
Radix Angelicae Sinensis	10g
Radix Paeoniae Alba	10g
Radix Codonopsis Philosulae	12g
Rhizoma Atractylodis Macrocephalae	10g
Poria	10g
Radix Curcumae	12g
Pericarpium Citri Reticulatae	10g
Radix Salviae Miltiorrhizae	12g
Rhizoma Dioscoreae	15g

Massa Fermentata Medicinalis	12g
Radix Glycyrrhizae Praeparata	6g

All the above drugs are to be decocted in water for oral aministration.

If the disease is characterized by dryness of the eyes, dizziness, dull pain in the hypochondrium, hot sensation in palms and soles, soreness and weakness in the loins and knees, dry and red tongue coated with a little fur or no fur at all, taut and thready pulse, which is caused by deficiency of the liver-yin, nourishing the liver-yin should dominates the treatment. The given recipe is Decoction for Nourishing the Liver and Kidney with additional ingredients:

Radix Glehniae	12g
Radix Ophiopogonis	12g
Radix Rehmanniae	12g
Fructus Lycii	15g
Radix Angelicae sinensis	10g
Fructus Meliae Toosendan	10g
Carapax Trionycis	15g
Radix Curcumae	12g
Herba Dendrobii	12g

(3) Stagnation of qi and blood stasis

Main symptoms and signs: Gloomy complexion, stabbing pain in the right hypochondrium, hepatomegaly or splenomegaly, abdominal distension, anorexia, some telangiectases in the skin of face and neck with vascular spiders, liver palms, dark purple tongue sometimes marked with ecchymoses, taut and uneven pulse.

Therapeutic principle: Promoting blood circulation, removing blood stasis and softening hard hepatomegaly or splenomegaly.

Recipe: Modified Decoction of Peach Kernel and Safflower with Other Four Ingredients.

Radix Angelicae Sinensis	12g
Radix Paeoniae Alba	12g
Rhizoma Ligustici Chuanxiong	10g
Semen Persicae	10g
Flos Carthami	10g
Radix Salviae Miltiorrhizae	20g

Carapax Trionycis	15g
Squama Manitis	6g
Rhizoma Zedoariae	10g
Caulis Spatholobi	30g
Rhizoma Cyperi	10g
Fructus Citri Sarcodactylis	10g
Radix Glycyrrhizae Praeparata	10g

All the above drugs are to be decocted in water for oral administration.

Apart from the above ingredients, 12 grams of dangshen (Radix Codonopsis Pilosulae) and 15 grams of astragalus root (Radix Astragali aeu Hedysari) are added for those with symptoms of lassitude and weakness.

For all types of clinical manifestations mentioned above, if SGPT is higher than normal, powder of schisandra fruit (Fructus Schisandrae) may be taken at the same time, 3 grams are taken each time and 3 times a day; or additional intake of stringy stonecrop powder (Herba Sedi Sarmentosi) 50 mg are taken each time and three times a day; or choose any of the appropriate amount of the following ingredients for extra intake: bistort rhizome (Rhizoma Bistortae), giant knotweed rhizome (Rhizoma Polygoni Cuspidati) and Japanese St. Johns wort (Herba Hyperici Japonici).

V ACUPUNCTURE AND MOXIBUSTION

Main points: Insert needles at Ganshu (BL 18), Danshu (BL 19), Pishu (BL 20), Zusanli (ST 36) and Zhiyang (DU 9) points to regulate the flow of qi in the liver and gallbladder and strengthen the function of spleen.

Supplementary points:

1) For cases with accumulation of damp-heat, add Yanglingquan (GB 34), Taichong (LR 3), Dazhui (DU 14) and Jianshi (PC 5) to eliminate damp-heat from the liver and gallbladder.

2) For cases with accumulation of cold-damp, perform needling and moxibustion at Yanggang (BL 48), Yinlingquan (SP 9) and Sanyinjiao (SP 6) to warm the spleen and eliminate dampness.

3) For cases with deficiency of yin, add Taichong (LR 3) and Taixi (KI 3)

to nourish yin of the liver and Kidneys.

4) For cases with stagnation of qi and blood stasis, add Taichong(LR 3), Qiuau(GB 40) and Geshu(BL 17) to regulate liver and gallbladder qi, promote blood circulation and remove stasis.

VI MEDICATED DIET

1) Gruel with Oriental Wormwood (Yinchen Zhou)

INGREDIENTS

Herba Artemisae Capillaris	30 to 45g
Semen Oryzae Sativae	100g
White sugar	a bit

PROCESS Have some oriental wormwood washed clean and use 30 to 45g at a time; add 200ml of water and decoct it until 100 ml of water is left. Remove the dregs to get the extract; put in 100g of polished round-grained rice, add 600 ml of water and cook until the rice is well-done and the extract becomes thick. Add a bit of white sugat and go on cooking for a while until it has boiled for a little while.

DIRECTIONS Take it 2 or 3 times a day, with 7 to 10 days as a course of treatment. It can be applied to acute icterohepatitis marked by the type of bile oozing from the gallbladder due to damp-heat accumulating in the liver and gallbladder.

2) Recipe of giant knotweed rhizome and honey (Huzhang mi)

INGREDIENTS

Rhizoma Polygoni Cuspitati	500g
Fructus schisandrae	250g
Mel	1000g

PROCESS Wash the giant knotweed rhizome and schisandra fruit clean, put them in an earthenware pot and add water (to the point that the two drugs can be submerged) and soak them for half an hour. Heat them over a moderate fire until the water boils. Then, change to a low fire and go on decocting for about half an hour until 500 ml of medicinal extract is left; filter it to get the extract. Add 1000 ml of water and heat it to get extract of about 500 ml; remove the dregs and put all the extract obtained and the honey into a big earthenware pot which is to be heated over a low fire. Let the decoction boil for 5 minutes, take the pot away from the fire to let it cool. Pour the decoction in a bottle and cover it tight.

DIRECTIONS Take a spoonful at a time after meals, three times a day after infusing it with boiling water, with two months as a course of treatment.

3) Decoction of oriental wormwood, germinated barley and jujube (Yinchen maiya hongzao tang)

INGREDIENTS

Herba Artemisiae Capillaris	15g
Fructus Hordei Germinatus	20g
Fructus Ziziphi Jujubae	10g
White sugar	a bit

PROGESS Put the oriental wormwood, germinated barley and jujubes in a small aluminium pan, add 1000 ml of cold water to stew the drugs slowly over a low fire for about half an hour; put in a half spoonful of white sugar and take in away from the fire.

DIRECTIONS Take less than half a bowlful at a time, twice a day. Drink the decoction, eat the jujubes and discard the dregs.

The above composite recipes are applicable to both the type of incoordination between the liver and the stomach caused by damp-heat accumulating in the interior, and the type of stagnancy of qi and blood in acute and chronic hepatitis. It can be used as an auxiliary treatment for chronic hepatitis patients.

4) Recipe of day lily and loach (Jinzhen niqiu)

INGREDIENTS

Flos Hemerocalis Immaturus	30g
Misgurnus Anguillicaudatus	100g

PROCESS Make soup with the day lily and loach flesh and season it for eating.

5) Drink of willow leaf and water chestnut (Liuye biqi cha)

INGREDIENTS

Folium Salicis	6g
Bulbus Heleocharis Tuberosae	500g

PROCESS Make decoction with 6 g of willow leaves and 500 g of water chestnuts.

DIRECTIONS Drink the decoction and eat the water chestnuts; take a dose a day, and several doses successively.

6) Recipe of canton love-pea vine and lean pork (Jigucao shouzhurou fang)

INGREDIENTS

Herba Abri	60g
Lean pork	100g

PROCESS Boil 100g of Canton love-pea vine and 100g of lean pork in just the right amount of water for two to three hours, remove the dregs and have it seasoned.

DIRECTIONS Take a dose once a day, for several days.

7) Loach and bean-curd (Niqiu cuan doufu)

INGREDIENTS

Bean-curd	100g
Misgurnus Anguillicaudatus	250g
Stigma Maydis (wrapped up in cloth)	30g

PROCESS Have the loach raised in a basin for 1 to 2 days; take it out and put it in an earthenware pot together with the corn stigma and bean-curd; add just the rignt amout of water to have them decocted. When they are thoroughly done, have them seasoned for eating.

DIRECTIONS Take it once a day, for sevral days.

8) Decoction of watermelon peel and red bean (Xiguapi chixiaodou tang)

INGREDIENTS

Exocarpium Citrulli	50g
Semen Phaseoli	50g
Rhizoma Imperatae	50g

PROCESS Make decoction with watermelon peel, red beans and cogongrass root.

DIRECTIONS Take the decoction once a day, for 5 to 7 days successively.

9) Celery stewed in honey (Mi dun qincai)

INGREDIENTS

Herba Apii	100 to 150g
Mel	right amount

PROCESS Have the celery washed clean and pounded into a mash to get the juice; stew the juice wijth honey.

DIRECTIONS Take the juice warm once a day, with no limit to the course of treatment.

10) Decoction of four "Red" Ingredients for tonifying the liver and eliminating dampness (Si hong yi gan li shi tang)

INGREDIENTS

Semen Phaseoli	60g
Semen Arachidis	30g
Fructus Ziziphi Jujubae	50g
Brown sugar	50g

PROCESS Put the red beans and peanut kernels in a pot after washing them clean, add 2000 ml of water to stew them slowly over a low fire for one and a half hours, then, put in the jujubes and brown sugar and go on stewing for about half an hour until the ingredients are thoroughly done.

DIRECTIONS Take a small bowlful of it as breakfast or snacks and take it twice a day.

11) Steamed soft-shelled turtle (Qingzheng jiayu)

INGREDIENTS

Trionyx Sinensis (weighing 200 to 300g)	1
Rhizoma Zingiberis Recens	3 slices
Refined salt	right amount
Millet wine	right amount

PROCESS Kill the soft-shelled turtle; soak it in boiling water to remove the membrane from the turtle, cut open its belly, remove its intestines and the like, retain the liver and the eggs that are still in the belly, wash it clean and drain the water out. Put the turtle in a porcelain basin with its back downward and put the ginger slices in its belly, spread the salt and sprinkle millet wine over it. Steam it without its contacting water over a brisk fire for 30 to 45 minutes.

DIRECTIONS Take it as light refreshments on an empty stomach, or take it with bread (or cooked rice). Any-way, take it hot. Being delicious, it has a great nutritive value and is a desirable therapeutic tonic for hepatitis patients and people of weak constitution.

12) Recipe of honey, sugar and soya-bean milk (Feng tang doujiang)

INGREDIENTS

    Lac Semi Sojae   a bowlful

    Mel   a spoonful

    White sugar   a bit

PROCESS Put a bowlful of saltless soya-bean milk, a spoonful of honey and a bit of white sugar into a small aluminium pan, then, heat it. Take the pan away from the fire as soon as the soya-bean milk has boiled.

DIRECTIONS Take it as breakfast with other light refreshments.

Chapter Four
Chronic Hepatitis

Chronic hepatitis is defined as a chronic inflammatory rection of the liver with a duration of over 6 months as demonstrated by persistently abnormal liver tests. For proper treatment, it is crucial to determine whether the disease will resolve, remain static, or progress to cirrhosis. The causes of chronic hepatits are only partially defined. It may be a sequela of infection resulting from hepatitis B virus. Chronic hepatitis has also been seen as a sequela of non-A, non—B hepatitis. Hepatitis A virus has not yet been shown to lead to chronic hepatitis.

1. Chronic persisting hepatitis

This form of chronic hepatitis represents and essentially benign condition with a good prognosis. The diagnosis is confirmed by liver biopsy. The biopsy may show portal tract infiltration with primarily mononuclear cells and occasional areas of focal inflammation in the parenchyma. The boundary between portal tracts and parenchyma remains sharp, and there is little or no "piecemeal necrosis."In essence, the architecture of the hepatic lobule remains intact. The symptomatology varies from the asymptomatic state to various vague manifestations including fatigability, anorexia, malaise and lassitude. Physical examination is usually normal.

Liver biopsy helps establish the diagnosis of persistent hepatitis. Treatment is mostly reassurance of the patient. Corticosteroids and immunosuppressive drugs should not be given. Dietary restrictions, excessive vitamin supplementation and prolonged bed rest are not necessary. The prognosis is excellent. Rarely does the disease progress to chronic active hepatitis.

2. Chronic active hepatitis (CAH)

This form of chronic hepatitis is usually characterized by progression to cirrhosis, although milder cases may resolve spontaneously. The histologic changes include chronic inflammatory infiltration involving portal zones and extending into the parenchyma, with piecemeal necrosis and the formation of intralobular septa. Piecemeal necrosis, a process of inflammatory cells and hepatocyte necrosis occurring at the interface of the portal area and the liver lobule, may extend well into the lobule and across zonal boundaries. In severe cases, piecemeal necrosis may be associated with considerable hepatic failure or fibrosis and ultimately with cirrhosis. In very mild cases, it may be difficult to distinguish this entity from chronic persistent hepatitis. Liver biopsies repeated at varying intervals may be necessary to make the distinction as well as to monitor therapy.

The disease is thought to be caused by internal stasis of dampness and heat in traditional Chinese medicine. The pathologic changes due to damp and heat pathogens stay deeply in the body. Thereby, various manifestations of gastrosplenic and cholehepatic dysfunctions may occur.

I CLINICAL MANIFESTATIONS

1. Symptoms and signs

A. Chronic persisting hepatitis. this is generally a disease of young people, particularly young women. However, the disease can occur at any age. The onset is usually insidious, but about 25% of cases present as an acute attack of hepatitis. Although the serum bilirubin is usually increased. 20% of these patients have anicteric disease. Examination often reveals a healthy-appearing young woman with multiple spider nevi, cutaneous striae, acne and hirsutism. Amenorrhea may be a feature of this disease. Multisystem involvement, including kidney, joints, lung and bowel and coombspositive hemolytic anemia are associated with this clinical entity.

B. Chronic active hepatitis (HBsAg -positive type). This type of hepatitis clinically resembles the lupoid type of disease. The histologic pictures of these two types of chronic active hepatitis are indistinguishable. The HBsAg form of chronic active hepatitis appears to affect males predominantly. It may be noted as a continuum of acute hepatitis or may be manifested only by biochemical abnormalities of liver function.

2. Laboratory findings

The serum bilirubin is usually normal or only modestly increased (4. 5-7mg/dL); SGOT(AST), IgG, IgM and gamma globulin levels are higher than normal. Late in the disease, serum albumin levels are usually decreased and prothrombin time may be significantly prolonged and will not respond to vitamin K therapy. Antinuclear and smooth muscle antibodies are positive 15-50% of the time. Latex fixation tests for rheumatoid arthritis and anticytoplasmic and immunofluorescent antimitochondrial antibodies are positive in 28-50% of patients. Hepatitis B antigen is not found in the blood of patients with classic"lupoid"hepatitis.

Activity in chronic liver disease can be defined quantitatively quite readily by establishing arbitrary biochemical standards. For example, either a 10-fold increase in serum transaminase level or a 5-fold elevation of SGOT with a 2-fold increase in gamma globulin concentration constitutes "high-grade"activity.

II MAIN POINTS OF DIAGNOSIS

Patients with chronic hepatitis may be entirely asymptomatic and exhibit only minimal abnormalities in routine laboratory tests, or may be incapacitated by progressive liver failure and the complications of portal hypertension. At any given time, the clinical and laboratory features may not correlate well with histopathology or long-term prognosis. For this reason and because concepts of the natural history and response to treatment are changing for some of these disorders, decisions regarding diagnosis, management and prognosis are often difficult and uncertain.

The concept of traditional Chinese medicine is that the stagnation of pathogenic damp and heat factors in the liver and the gallbladder influences and causes the spleen and stomach to become deficient. If this condition lasts for a long time, the stagnation of Qi and the depression of blood in the liver may occur.

III DIFFERENTIATION AND TREATMENT OF COMMON SYNDROMES

1. Classified this affction into five types.

1) Liver stasis. Liver stasis is a short term for the stagnation and depression of the hepatic Qi. When the dispersing function of the liver is disturbed, there may appear various symptoms such as fullness or burning pain of the hypochondrium, chest distress, mental depression or anxiety, feeling of a lump in the throat, occasional epigastric distension and pain, hiccup, regurgitation of acid, suppressed appetite, occasional abdominal distension and pain, diarrhea. The treatment is to cleat the liver with Xiao Yao san Jia Jian.

Recipe

Root of Chinese angelica	20g
Unpeeled root of herbaceous peony	30g
Root of herbaceous peony	30g
Chinese thorowax	15g
Tuckahoe	10g
Large-headed atractylodes	15g
Nutgrass flatsedge	15g
Root-tuber of aromatic turmeric	12g
Rhizoma corydalis	12g
Fruit of hawthorn	15g
Medicated leaven	30g
Malt	30g
Capillary artemisia	30g
Loosestrife	30g

Decoction and dosage: All the above herbs make a dose and six to ten doses are prescribed with one dose daily. Each dose is simmered twice and then the broth of each mixed, half of the mixed broth each time, twice a day.

2) The type due to the invasion of stomach by hepatic Qi. When the dispersing function of the liver is disturbed and the stomach is affected, there appear simultaneous pathologic manifestations of both the liver and the stomach. The main symptoms are vertigo, chest distress, hypochondriac pain, irritability and

excitability, epigastric distension and pain, anorexia, nausea and vomiting, regurgitation of acid, stringy pulse, etc. The principle of treatment is to cleat the-liver and strengthen the spleen. The commonly used formula is Chai Ping Yin Jia Jian.

Pecipe

Chinses thorowax	12g
Pinellia	12g
Dangshen	12g
Skullcap	10g
Chinese atractylodes	12g
Bark of official magnolia	12g
Dried old orange peel	12g
Rhizoma corydalis	15g
Fruit of citron or trifoliate orange	15g
Fruit of hawthorn	10g
Medicated leaven	15g
Malt	30g
Capillary artemisia	30g
Loosestrife	30g

Decoction and dosage is the same.

3) The type caused by depressed liver and insufficient spleen. When the dispersing function of the liver is disturbed and the spleen is affected, there appear simultaneously pathologic manifestations of the liver and the spleen. The main symptoms are vertigo, chest distress, hypochondriac pain, irritability and excitability, distension of the abdomen, loose stools, anorexia, stringy pulse, etc. The treatment is to strengthen the spleen and clear the liver with Qui Shao Liu Jun Zhi Tang Jia Jian.

Recipe

Root of Chinese angelica	30g
Unpeeled root of herbaceous peony	30g
Root of herbaceous	30g
Dangshen	15g
Large-headed atractylodes (baked)	30g
Tuckahoe	15g

Dried old orange peel	12g
Pinellia	12g
Job's tears	30g
Chinese yan rhizome	30g
Fruit of hawthorn	30g
Medicated leaven	30g
Malt	30g
Winkled gianthyssop	12g
Capillary artemisia	30g
Loosestrife	45g

Decoction and dosage is the asme.

4) The type due to substantial heat in the liver and the gallbladder. The pathologic changes are due to stagnation of pathogenic damp and heat factors in the liver and the gallbladder. The main symptoms are jaundice, fever, bitter taste, pain in the hypochodrium, nausea and vomiting, anorexia, aversion to fatty food, abdominal distension and pain, yellowish urine, loose stools, yellowish glossy coating of the tongue, stringy and rapid pulse, etc. The treatment is to cleat the heat and excrete the dampness with Yin Chen shi Lin Tang Jia Jian.

Recipe

Capillary artemisia	60g
Capejasmine	12g
Skullcap	10g
Loosestrife	60g
Tuckahoe	30g
Oriental water plantain	12g
Umbellate pore fungus	15g
Cogongrass rhizome	60g
Giant knotweek	30g
Fruit of hawthorn	12g
Medicated leaven	15g
Malt	15g
Rough gentian	15g

Decoction and dosage is the same.

5) The type due to stagnation of Qi and blood. The liver is enlarged, palpa-

ble, firm if not hard, and has a blunt edge. The skin manifestations consist of spider nevi (only on the upper half of the body), palmar erythema (mottled redness of thenar and hypothenar eminences). The treatment is to break the stagnant Qi and activate the blood with Fu Yuan Hou Xue Tang Jia Jian.

Recipe

Root of Chinese angelica	30g
Unpeeled root of herbaceous peony	30g
Chuanxiong	15g
Peach kernel	15g
Safflower	15g
Root of red rooted salvia	30g
Pangolinscale	10g
Rhubarb	6g
Chinese thorowax	12g
Nutgrass flatsedge	12g
Root-tuber of aromatic turmeric	12g
Zodoary turmeric	18g
Rhizoma corydalis	10g

Decoction and dosage is the same.

2. Classified this affection into three types.

1) Accumulation of damp due to spleen deficiency

Main symptoms and signs: Pain in the liver region, jaundice, dark yellow colour of the skin and sclera, poor appetite, fullness and distension of the abdomen, loose stool, fatigue and lassitude, tastelessness in the mouth. White, thick and greasy tongue coating, wiry and thready pulse.

Therapeutic principle: Warm yang and strengthen the spleen to expel the damp.

Recipe:

Ginseng	9g
White atractylodes rhizome	15g
Poria	15g
Coix seed	30g
Tangerine peel	9g
Prepared aconite root	40g

Orlental wormwood	30g
Hawthorn fruit	9g
Malt	9g
Medicated leaven	9g

Decocted in water for oral administration

External treatment: Hepatitis-recovering and Umbilicus-treating Belt (Gan-fukang Qiliao Dai) is tightened along the umbilical region.

(2) Deficiency of the liver yin

Main symptoms and signs: Dull pain in the hypochodrium, dryness of eyes, dizziness, blurred vision, hot sensation in the palms and soles, soreness and weakness in the loins and knees. Dry and red tongue with little or no coating, wiry and thready pulse.

Therapeutic principle: Nourish the liver yin.

Recipe:

Dried rehmannia root	30g
Glehnia root	15g
Ophiopogon root	15g
Wolfberry fruit	15g
Chinese angelica root	12g
Sichuan chinaberry	12g
Fresh-water turtle shell	15g
Curcuman root	12g
Dendrobium stem	12g

Decocted in water for oral administration

Patent medicine: Liver-tonic-infusion of Versicolor (Yunzhi Gantai Chongji). Take 10g each time, 3 times a day.

(3) Liver qi stagnation

Main symptoms and sings: stabbing pain in the right hypochondrium, lumps in the hypochondrium, abdominal distension, anorexia, dark complexion, restlessness, irritability, liver palms. Dark tongue with ecchymoses, wiry and hesitant pulse.

Therapeutic principle: Soothe the liver and regulate qi, activate the blood and disperse stasis.

Recipe:

Bupleurum root	9g
Chinses angelica root	12g
White peony root	15g
White atractylodes rhizome	12g
Poria	12g
Tangerine peel	9g
Curcuma root	9g
Red asge root	30g
Peach kernel	9g
Safflower	9g
Fresh-water turtle shell	15g
Pangolin scales	6g
Spatholobus stem	30g
Cyperus tuber	9g
Finger citron	9g
Prepared licorice root	9g

Decocted in water for oral administration

Patent medicine: Liver-restoring Tablet (Liganlong Pian). Take 5 tablets each time, 3 times a day.

IV ACUPUNCTURE AND MOXIGUSTION

1. Body acupuncture

1) Points: Yanglingquan(BL 34), Zhigou(ST 6) and Qimen(LR 14).

Method: All the points are punctured with reducing method. But for patients with stagnation of Qi, Ganshu(BL 18) and Qiuxu(BL 40) are added to the prescription and for patients with stagnation of blood, Geshu(BL 17) and Xingjian(LR 2) are included.

2) Main Points: Ganshu (BL18) and Danshu (BL19).

Supplementary Points: Add Pishu (BL20), Zhiyang (DU 9), Zhongwan (RN12), Zusanli(ST36) and Sanyinjiao (SP6) for jaundice (yin jaundice); add Yanglingquan (GB34), Taichong(LR3) and Xuehai (SP10) for stagnation of qi and blood staisis.

Needling method: Use the filiform needles with even movement.

2. Ear-acupuncture therapy.

Points: Chest Pt, Ear-shemen Pt and Liver Pt.

Method: Select 2 to 3 points on the affected side of the ear and puncture with the needles ratained for 20 to 30 minutes.

3. Point injection

Points: Ganshu (BL18), Pishu (BL20) and Zhongdu (LR6).

Method: The Isatis Injection, Salvia Injection or vit B_1, Vit. B_{12} Injection are advisable. 0. 5 to 1 ml would be injected into each point. 2 points are used each treatment. The treatment is given onceevery other day. 10 treatments make a course.

V   MEDICATED DIET

1. Stew red bean 60g and peanut kernel 30g in 2000 ml of water over a low fire for 1. 5 hours after washing them clean. Then put jujube 10 pieces and brown sugar 50g in it and go on stewing for about 0. 5 hour until the ingredients are thoroughly done. Take a small bowlful each time, twice a day.

2. Stew orietal wormwood 15g, germinated barley 21g and jujube 10 pieces in 1000 ml of cold water slowly over a low fire for about 0. 5 hour. Then put a little of white sugar in it and take it from the fire. Take less than half a bowlful each time, twice a day. Drink the decoction, eat the jujubes and discard the dregs.

3. Kill a soft-shelled turtle. Soak it in boiling water to remove the membrane from the turtle. Cut open its belly; remove its intestines and the likes; ratain the liver and the eggs; wash it clean and drain the water out. Put the turtle in a porcelain basin with its back downward and put 3 slices of fresh ginger inside its belly. Spread right amount of salt and sprinkle rice wine over it. Steam it over boiling water with a high flame fire for 30 to 40 minutes. Take it hot as refreshments or with rice.

Chapter Five
Hepatocirrhosis

Hepatocirrhosis is the final outcome of diffuse inflammation of the liver, degeneration and necrosis of the hepatic cells and proliferation of fibrous tissue induced by various causes. Of the causes of the disease, posthepatitic cirrhosis is the most common one, second ones are the cardiac, biliary and alcoholic cirrhosis. Nodular cirrhosis is closely related to liver carcinoma.

In TCM, hepatocirrhosis (HC) belongs to the categories of "Stagnation of liver qi"(gan yu), "hepatosplenomegaly"(pi kuai), " Mass in the abdomen" (zheng ji), " tympanites"(gu zhang) etc. According to symptom-sign differentiation, it is ascribed to deficiency in the base and excessiveness in the superficies. It is often caused by the impairment of the liver, spleen and kidney and the accumulation of Qi, blood and water. The general treatment regimen for HC calls for the elimination of blood stasis and the regulation of Qi, the softening of solids and the dissipation of mass, the excretion of dampness and the draining of water, and finally the attending to the improvement of patient's resistance. In clinical practice, these above mentioned principles can be dealt with flexibly depending on the condition of deficiency and excessiveness as well as the tendency of the impaired viscera.

I CLASIFICATION

1. Micronodular (portal cirrhosis) is characterised by regulat thick fibrotic bands joining the portal tracts to hepatic veins, and with small regenerative nodules. The liver is initially large with a smooth edge but subsequently shrinks with progressive fibrosis. It is often alcoholic in origin and is then associated with fatty infiltration.

2. Macronodular (post-necrotic cirrhosis) is less common and is characterised by course, irregular bands of fibrosis and loss of normal architecture and large regenerative nodules. It is believed usually to follow viral hepatitis with widespread necrosis.

3. Biliary cirrhosis is less common and is characterised by fibrosis around

distended intrahepatic bile ducts. It may follow chronic cholangitis and biliary obstruction (secondary), or be idiopathic (primary).

4. Cardiac cirrhosis may occur in chronic cardiac failure. Centrilobular congestion leads to necrosis and fibrosis, but nodular regeneration is not marked.

5. Other rare causes of cirrhosis include chronic aggressive hepatitis, haemochromatosis and hepatolenticular degeneration.

II MAIN POINTS OF DIAGNOSIS

1. Compensatory Phase: Clinical manifestations include fatigue, loss of appetite, nausea, abdominal fullness and other symptoms of digestive tract. Slight edema and bleeding tendency may be present due to reduced liver function. The findings of physical examination are mild hepatomegaly with slight hardness, spleneomegal, spider nevi and liver palms.

2. Decompensatory Phase

(1) Portal hypertension syndrome: Splenomegaly with hypersplenism, esophageal and gastric fundal venous varices which may result in hemorrhage of the upper digestive tract.

(2) Impaired liver function syndrome: Fatigue and symptoms of the digestive tract are aggravated, low fever, jaundice, edema and ascites are often present. Patients may have eminent bleeding tendency, darkish complexion and endocrine disorder. In severe cases complications such as hemorrhage of the upper digestive tract and hepatic coma may take their place.

3. Laboratory examination

(1) Liver function test: It is found that icteric index has increased, A/G ratio decreased or reversed, γ-globulin increased. Flocculation-turbidity test presents a positive; SGPT, transpeptidase and MAO, too elevated. The prothrombin time is often elongated.

(2) Ultrasonography (A and B Mode), liver scan, CT scanning and liver puncture are helpful in confirming the diagnosis and type of the disease. They are also valuable in differentiation from other liver disease such as hepatic carcinoma and liver abscess.

IⅡ DIFFERENTIATION AND
TREATMENT OF COMMON SYNDROMES

1. Stagnation of the liver-qi and deficiency of the spleen

Main symptoms and signs: Anorexi, abdominal distress and distension, vague hypochondriac pain, lassitude and fatigue, or nausesa and loose stool, whitish coating of the tongue, and taut pulse.

Therapeutic principle: Relieving the depressed liver-qi and invigorating the spleen, promoting blood circulation to remove blood stasis.

Recipe: Modified Ease Powder.

Radix Bupleuri	12g
Radix Angelicae Sinensis	15g
Radix Paeoniae Alba	15g
Rhizoma Atractylodis Macrocephalae	15g
Poria	9g
Rhizoma Cyperi	9g
Fructus Citri Sarcodactylis	12g
Radix Salviae Miltiorrhizae	15g
Endothelium Corneum Gigeriae Galli	9g
Radix Glycyrrhizae Preaparata	6g

All the above drugs are to be decocted in water for oral administration.

Besides, 10 grams of atractylodes rhizome (Rhizoma Atracrtylodis) and 10 grams of magnoslia bark (Cortex Magnoliae Officinalis) ought to be administered for the case with thick coating of the tongue and distension of the abdomen due to abundance of pathogenic dampness; 12 grams of dangshen(Radix Codonopsis Pilosulae) and 12 grams of wolfberry fruit (Fructus Lycii) administered for the case with obvious fatigue.

2. Obstruction of the liver-blood

Main symptoms and sings: Hepatomegaly and splemomegaly, twinge or distress in the hypochondrium, distension of the abdomen, anorexia, dim complexion, or accompanied with spider nevi and liver palms, deep-red tongue or with ecchymoses, taut and thready pulse.

Therapeutic principle: Promoting blood circulation to remove blood stasis, softening hard hepatosplenomegaly to remove obstruction in the liver-channel.

Recipe: Modified Decoction for Removing blood Stasis.

Radix Angelicae Sinensis	12g
Radix Salviae Miltiorrhizae	15g
Semen Persicae	10g
Flos Carthami	10g
Radix Curcumae	10g
Radix Bupleuri	10g
Pericarpium Citri Reticulatea Viride	10g
Carapex Trionycis	15g
Squama Manitis	10g
Concha ostreae	30g
Rhizoma Atractylodis Macrocephalae	12g
Radix Glycyrrhizae Praeparata	6g

In addition, the administration of dangshen (Radix Codonopsis Pilosulae) 12g and astragalus root (Radix Astragali seu Hedysari) 15g is for patients with symptoms of deficiency of qi; dried rehmannia root (Radix Rehmanniae) 12g and dendrobium (Herba Dendrobii) 10g for patients with manifestations of impairment of yin.

3. Retention of water within the body

Main symptoms and signs: Tympanites which is firm and full when pressed, epigastric distress, anorexia, scanty urine, red tongue, taut and thready pulse.

Therapeutic principle: Regulating the flow of qi to induce diuresis, removing blood stasis to soften hard hepatosplenomigaly.

Recipe: Modified Stomach Decoction with Poria.

Rhizoma Atractylodis	10g
Rhizoma Atractylodis Macrocephalae	10g
Cortex Magnoliae Officinalis	10g
Poria	15g
Polyporus Umbellatus	12g
Rhizoma Alismatis	15g
Pericarpium Arecae	15g

Semen Plantaginis （wrapped in a piece of cloth for decoction）

	20g
Radix Aucklandiae	10g
Radix salviae Miltiorrhizae	15g
Carapax Trionycis	15g
Semen Persicae	10g
Radix Glycyrrhizae Praeparata	6g

All the above drugs are to be decocted in water for oral administration.

If the case is complicated with deficiency of the liver-yin and kidney-yin marked by abdominal distension with dry mouth and lips, hot sensation in the palms and soles, deep-red tongue with very little fur or none, and taut, thready and rapid pulse, the treatment should be concentrated on nourishing the liver and kidney, and nourishing yin and inducing diuresis. The modified Decoction for Nourishing the Liver and Kidney is preferable for the very treatment. The compositions are: glehnia root （Radix Glehniae ）,10g ophiopogon root（Radix Ophiopogonis） 10g, dried rehmannia root （Radix rehmanniae） 15g, wolfberry fruit （Fructus Lycii)12g, umbellate pore-fungus （Polyporus Umblelatus)15g, water-plantain tuber （Rhizoma Alismatis） 15g, poria （Poria） 15g, tale （Talcum） 12g, oyster shell （Concha Ostreae)30g, red sage root （Radix Salviae Miltiorrhizae） 15g, fresh-water turtle shell(Carapax Trionycis) 15g. All the drugs are to be decocted in water for oral administration.

Yao Changli divided this disease into seven types:

1. Gathering and brewing of dampness and heat within the body.

Main symptons and signs: Rapid appearance of ascitic fluid, tympanites which is lustrous and cann't be pressed, yellow discoloration of sclera and skin, poor appetite, thirst, but no desire to drink much water, dark yellowish and scanty urine, constipation or loose stool with offensive odour and uncomfortable feeling while defecating, crimson tongue with greasy or grey-dark coating, thickened and dark-purplish sublingual veins with yellow discoloration of the small blood vessels, rapid, taut and slippery pulse or rapid and soft pulse.

Recipe:

Herba Artemisiae Capillaris	10g
Radix Gentianae Macrophyllae	10g
Fructus Gardeniae	10g

Radix et Rhizoma Rhei	10g
Talcum	10g
Pericarpium Arecae	10g
Pericarpium Poria	10g
Polyporus Umbellatus	10g
Rhizoma Alismatis	10g
Exocarpium Benincasae	10g
Semen Plantaginis	10g
Rhizoma Imperatae	10g

2. Obstruction of qi due to depression of liver

Main symptoms and signs: Sensation of swelling and fullness in the abdomen which is not hard when palpated, sensation of hypochondriac swelling and pain which is slightly relieved after belching or passing gas, little appetite, acanty urine, loose stool with little amount but increased frequency of bowel novement, dark-red tongue with white coating or thin-yellowish greasy coating, blue-purplish and thickened sublingual veins, soft or taut-slippery pulse.

Recipe:

Radix Bupleuri	10g
Fructus Aurantii	10g
Radix Paeoniae Rubra	10g
Radix Paeoniae Alba	10g
Radix Curcurae	10g
Rhizoma Polygoni Cuspidati	10g
Retinervus	10g
Fructus Luffae	10g
Pericarpium Poria	10g
Rhizoma Alismatis	10g
Polyporus Umbellatus	10g
Exocarpium Benincasae	10g
Semen Coicis	10g
Radix Salviae Miltiorrhizae	10g
Radix Ophiopogonis	10g
Fructus Chaenomelis	10g
Radix Glycyrrhizae	10g

3. Blood stasis and water retention

Main symptoms and signs: Tympanites which is firm and full while palpated, varicosis in abdominal wall, hypochondriac mass with twing, spider nevi seen in the neck and the chest; liver palms sometimes accompanied by chaffy and dry skin; yellowish and scanty urine; loose stool, or in dark grey color; dark-purplish togue with ecchymoses, thin-white or slightly yellow coating, deep-uneven or taut-uneven forceful pulse.

Recipe:

Radix Angelicae Sinensis	10g
Semen Persicae	10g
Radix Salviae Miltiorrhizae	10g
Radix Paeoniae Rubra	10g
Radix Paeoniae Alba	10g
Radix Curcumae	10g
Radix Notoginseng (ground to powder)	10g
Rhizoma Polygoni Cuspidati	10g
Pericarpium Arecae	10g
Pericarpium Poria	10g
Rhizoma Alismatis	10g
Polyporus Umbellatus	10g
Exocarpium Benincasae	10g
Radix Ophiopogonis	10g
Radix Glycyrrhizae	10g

4. Retention of dampness due to spleen deficiency

Main symptoms and signs: Sallow complexion, lassitude and disinclination to talk, swelling of the abdomen which is soft while palpated and worsened after eating, poor appetite, scanty urine and loose stool, dropsy in the legs, plump tongue with light dark color and tooth marks on its edges, thin-white or white-greasy coating, light purplish sublingual veins, thin-slippery or taut-slippery pulse.

Recipe:

Rhizoma Atractylodis Macrocephalae	10g
Semen Coicis	10g
Radix Aconiti Lateralis praeparata	10g

Radix Achyranthis Bidentatae	10g
Pericarpium Citri Reticulatae	10g
Semen Alpiniae Katsumadai	10g
Pericarpium Arecae	10g
Semen Plantaginis	10g
Pericarpium Poria	10g
Rhizoma Alismatis	10g
Polyporus Umbellatus	10g
Exocarpium Benincasae	10g
Radix Aucklandiae	10g
Radix Ophiopogonis	10g
Radix Glycyrrhizae.	10g

5. Yang deficiency in the spleen and kidney

Main symptoms and signs: pale complexion, chills, cold limbs, listless waist and legs, shortness of breath, disinclination to talk, tympanite like the abdomen of a frog which worsens at night, scanty urine, loose stool, dropsy in the legs, plump but tender tongue of pale and dark color, accompanied by tooth marks on its edge, thin coating, slender and forceless pulse.

Recipe:

Radix Codonopsis Pilosulae	10g
Rhizoma Atractylodis Macrocephalae	10g
Semen Coicis	10g
Fructus Corni	10g
Semen Cuscutae	10g
Fructus Psoraleae	10g
Radix Aconiti Lateralis Praeparata	10g
Ramulus Cinnamomi	10g
Radix Achyranthis Bidentatae	10g
Pericarpium Poria	10g
Rhizoma Alismatis	10g
Polyporus Umbellatus	10g
Semen Plantaginis	10g
Exocarpium Benincasae	10g
Radix Glycyrrhizae	10g

6. Deficiency of both qi and yin

Main symptoms and signs: Lustreless complexion, red cheeks in the afternoon, lassitude and weakness, shortness of breath and weak voice, burning sensation in the palme and soles, tympanite with varicosis in the abdominal wall, scanty urine, dry stool first, then loose stool, dry mouth and throat, but no desire to drink much water, slightly dropsical legs, red tongue with cracks on it, scant coating; slender, soft and forceless pulse.

Recipe:

Radix Astragali seu Hedysari	30g
Radix Angelicae Sinensis	30g
Radix Codonopsis Pilosulae	30g
Radix Glehniae	15g
Radix Ophiopogonis	15g
Semen Coicis	10g
Fructus Schisandrae Semen Plantaginis	10g
Radix achyranthis bidentatae	10g
Pericarpium Poria	10g
Rhizoma Alismatis	10g
Polyporus Umbellatus	10g
Exocarpium Benincasea	10g
Pericarpium Lagenariae (state)	10g
Herba Aristolochiae	10g
Radix Glycyrrhizae	10g.

7. Yin deficiency of liver and kidney.

Main symptoms and signs: Dark and soiled complexion, spider nevi and blood streaks on the face, neck and chest, obvious liver palms, emaciation, tympanite with varicosis, chaffy and dry skin, dizziness and blurred eyes, dysphoria and poor sleep, recurred fever, bloody nose or gums, dry mouth and teeth, scanty urine with foul odour, loose stool like duck's; red, mirror-like tongue, or with cracks, pricks on the edge and tip of the tongue, little or no coating, thin-rapid or taut -thin pulse.

Recipe:

Radix Glehniae	20g
Radix Ophiopogonis	20g

Radix Rehmanniae	20g
Fructus Lycii	10g
Rhizoma Polygonati	10g
Colla Corii Asini	10g
Colla Plastri Testudinis	10g
Semen Plantaginis	10g
Radix Achyranthis Bidentatae	10g
Retinervus Luffae Fructus	10g
Rhizoma Alismatis	10g
Radix Glycyrrhizae	10g
Pericarpium Lagenariae	10g
Pericarpium Citri Reticulatae	10g

163 cases were treated with the above method. 59 cases were cured. 30 cases improved considerably. 34 cases partially improved. The overall effectiveness of treatment was rated at 79.1%.

IV THERAPEUTIC METHODS OF CHINESE QIGONG

1. Self-treatment by practising qigong

1) Basic maneuvers

Practise Heavenly Circuit Self-Roatation Qigong, Inner-nourishing Qigong and Eight-section Brocade.

2) Auxiliary maneuvers

(1) Stagnation of the liver-qi and deficiency of the spleen: It is advisable to practise the methods of pushing and conducting to regulate the flow of qi and rubbing the costal region to send down abnormally ascending qi in Sternocostal Qigong.

(2) Stagnancy of qi and blood stasis: It is advisable to practise the methods of rubbing the chest and training qi with the word "xu"as well as soothing the liver and conducting qi in Regulating-liver qigong.

(3) Retention of water within the body: It is advisable to practise the methods of rubbing the epigastrium and training qi with the word "hu"as well as dredging the spleen and the stomach in Regulating-spleen Qigong. Those with

insufficiency of the spleen-yang and kidney-yang are advised to practise Gathering Sun Essence Qigong; those with deficiency of the liver-yin and kidney-yin are advised to practise Gathering Moon Cream Qigong.

2. External qi (Waiqi) therapy

1) Basic maneuvers

(1) First tip and knead the acupoints Ganshu (Liver shu, BL 18), Pishu (Spleen shu, BL 20), Zhongwan (Widdle Epigastrium, RN 12), Zhangmen (Bright Door, LR 13) and Qimen (Cyclic Door, LR 14).

(2) Apply the flat-palm form, use the vibrating and quivering manipulations to emit qi onto Zhongwan (Middle Epigastrium, RN 12), Qimen (Cyclic Door, LR 14), Ganshu (Liver shu, BL 18) and Pishu (Spleen shu , BL 20) for 14 or 28 breaths respectively.

(3) Apply the flat-palm form, use the pushing, pulling and leading manipulations to emit qi onto Ganshu (Liver Shu, BL 18), Qimen (Cyclic door, LR 14) and Zhangmen (Bright Door, LR 13), and conduct qi downward along the Gall Bladder Channel and the Liver Channel.

2) Auxiliary maneuvers

(1) Stagnation of the liver-qi and deficiency of the spleen: Apply the middle-finger standing-alone form, use the vibrating and quivering manipulations to emit qi onto Pishu (Spleen shu, BL 20) and Zhongwan (Middle Epigastrium, RN 12).

(2) Stagnancy of qi and blood stasis: Apply the flat-palm form, use the pulling and leading manipulations to emit qi onto Qimen (Cyclic Door, LR 14) and Zhangmen (Bright Door, LR 13), and conduct qi along the Gall Bladder Channel down to the acupoint Yanglingquan (Yang Mound Spring, GB 34) on the lower limbs.

(3) Retention of water within the body: Apply the flat-palm form, use the pulling and leading manipulations to emit qi onto Dabao (General Control, SP 21), and conduct qi along the spleen Channel to the lower limbs. Those with either insuffciency of the splecn-yang and kidney-yang or deficiency of the liver-yin and kidney-yin are advised to apply the middle-finger standing-alone form and use the vibrating and quivering manipulations to emit qi onto Guanyuan (Energy Pass, RN 4), Shenshu (Kidney Shu, BL 23) and Pishu (Spleen Shu, BL 20).

V MEDICATED DIET

1) Peach kernel gruel with additions (Fufang taoren zhou)

INGREDIENTS

Semen Persicae	9g
Pericarpium Citri Reticulatae	6g
Fructus Crataegi	12g
Semen Oryzae Sativae	100g

PROCESS Decoct the first threee ingredients in water, remove the dregs from the decoction; then add the rice and a right amount of water to the decoction and cook them into gruel.

DIRECTIONS To be taken twice each day for the treatment of early cirrhosis belonging to stagnation of qi and blood stasis.

2) Soup of pork stewed with dangshen and astragalus root with additions (Fufang shen qi zhurou tang)

INGREDIENTS

Radix Codonopsis Pilosulae	12g
Radix Astragali seu Hedysari	12g
Poria	12g
Rhizoma Atractylodis Macrocephalae	9g
Ganoderma Lucidum	6g
Pericarpium Citri Reticulatae	6g
Fructus Citri Sarcodactylis	6g
Fructus Amomi	3g
Lean Pork	100g
Bulbus Allii Fistulosi	right amount
Rhizoma Zingiberis Recens	right amount
Soy sauce and table salt	right amount

PROCESS Stew the pork with all the ingredients and a right amount of water over slow fire until the pork is well-done.

DIRECTIONS The meat is to be eaten and the soup to be drunk. It is applicable to patients suffering from early cirrhosis belonging to stagnation of the liver-qi and deficiency of the spleen.

3) Soup of turtle stewed with chinese angelica root and wolfberry friit (Gui qi jiayu tang)

INGREDIENTS

Radix Angelicae Sinensis	9g
Fructus Lycii	9g
Radix Rehmanniae praeparata	6g
Radix Ophiopogonis	6g
Fructus Ligustri Lucidi	6g
Rhizoma Dioscoreae	6g
Pericarpium Citri Reticulatae	6g
Amyda Sinensis	1
Bulbus Allii Fistulosi	right amount
Rhizoma Zingiberis Recens	right amount

PROCESS Put the first seven ingredients in a gauze bag; kill the turtle, cut it open, clean it of the entrails and wash it clean; place the gauze bag of drugs into the body cavity of the turtle, put turtle in an earthenware pot, pour in a right amount of water and the seasonings. Stew the turtle with slow fire until it is well-done and then take out the bag of drugs.

DIRECTIONS The turtle is for eating and the soup for drinking. It is applicable to early cirrhosis manifested as the syndrome of deficfiency of yin.

4) Gruel of citron fruit, finger citron and radish seed (Xiang fo laifu zhou)

INGREDIENTS

Fructus Citri	9g
Fructus Citri Sarcodactylis	9g
Semen Raphani (groud into powder)	15g
Semen Oryzae Sativae	100g

PROCESS Decoct the first two ingredients in water, remove the dregs from the decoction; then add to the decoction the radish seed powder, the rice and a right amount of water and make them into gruel.

DIRECTIONS To be taken twice on the same day. Applicable to cirrhosis manifested as tympanites due to stagnation of qi.

5) Soup of carp inducing diuresis (Lishui liyu tang)

INGREDIENTS

Cyprinus Carpio(about 250 to 500g)	1

Stigma Maydis	30g
Semen Phaseoli	30g
Exocarpium Benincasae	15g
Poria	15g
Polyporus	15g
Rhizoma Alismatis	15g
Pericarpium citri Reticulatae	6g
Bulbus Allii Fistulosi	right amount
Rhizoma Zingiberis Recens	right amount

PROCESS First get rid of the scales of the carp, remove its entrails, wash it clean and place it in an earthenware pot; then put all the other ingredients into the pot with a right amount of water; after all this having been done, stew it with slow fire until the fish is well-done.

DIRECTIONS The fish is to be eaten and the soup to be drunk. Applicable to ascites due to cirrhosis.

6) Gruel of red peony root, peach kernel, Chinese angelica root and poria (Chi tao gui ling zhou)

INGREDIENTS

Radix Paeoniae Rubra	9g
Semen Persicae	9g
Radix Angelicae Sinensis	9g
Fructus Polygoni Orientalis	6g
Pericarpium Citri Reticulatae	6g
Poria	12g
Polyporus	12g
Semen Phaseoli	30g
Semen Oryzae Sativae	60g

PROCESS Decoct the first seven ingredients in water, remove the dregs from the decoction; then add in the red phaseolus bean, the rice and a right amount of water and make them into gruel.

DIRECTIONS To be taken twice each day. Applicable to cirrhosis manifested as the symptoms of tympanites due to blood stasis.

7) Finger citron and rose tea (Fo hua cha)

INGREDIENTS

| Fructus Citri Sarcodactylis | 9g |
| Flos rosae Rugosae | 6g |

PROCESS Infuse them in boiling water.

DIRECTIONS To be taken as a drink. Its indications are the same as those of Activating qi and Promoting Digestion and Drink of Tangerine Peel with Additions.

8) Composite drink of corn stigma (Fufang yumixu yin)

INGREDIENTS

Stigma Maydis	30g
Exocarpium Benincasae	15g
Pericarpium Poriae	15g

PROCESS Decoct all the three ingredients in water and sift the decoction from the dregs.

DIRECTIONS To be taken as a daily drink.

9) Composite gruel of red phaseolus bean (Fufang chidou zhou)

INGREDIENTS

Semen Phaseoli	30g
Semen Coicis	30g
Semen Oryzae Sativae	30g
Pericarpium Citri Reticulatae	3g

PROCESS Make gruel with all the four ingredients.

DIRECTIONS To be taken twice on the same day. It has the same indications as Soup of Carp Inducing Diuresis.

10) Gruel activating qi and promoting digestion (Xingqi jianwei zhou).

11) Drink of tangerine peel with additions (Fufang jupi cha).

For these two recipes, refer to Chronic Gastritis; they are used to treat cirrhosis belonging to stagnation of qi.

Chapter Six
Cholecystitish

Acute cholecystitis is caused mainly by bacterial infection and biliary tract obstruction; chronic cholecystitis usually coexists with gallstone besides a history of acute cholecystitis. In TCM, this disease is categorized as "xie tong" (hypochondriac pain), "huang dan" (jaundice), etc.

I ACUTE CHOLECYSTITIS

Clinical features

The story is of fever, occasionally with rigors, abdominal pain. Usually right subcostal with acute pain on palpation over the gall bladder region. The disease is more common in obese females over 50, but may occur in young adults. Gall-stones are present in over 90% of cases. Occasionally, acute cholecystitis may be difficult to distinguish from a high appendix and right basal pneumonia and even perforated peptic ulcer, pancreatitis and myocardial infection.

Management

The acute inflammation usually settles with bed rest, analgesia (pethidine) and antibiotics. Ampicillin and cotrimoxazole are both secreted in the bile. Rarely, an empyema develops or the gall bladder perforates.

II CHRONIC CHOLECYSTITIS

Recurrent episodes of cholecystitis are usually associated with gallstones (more than 90%). The attacks are often less severe than classical acute cholecystitis, and may resemble peptic ulceration and peptic oesophagitis. Myocardial ischaemia may be confused if the site of the pain is high.

III GALL-STONES

Twice as common in women as men. The incidence rises with age. Stones occur in 10% of women over 40. They are usually cholesterol or mixed. Rarely they are pigment stones associated with haemolytic anaemia.

Clinical features

Most stones produce no symptoms, but they may cause: Flatulence up Biliary colic, acute cholecystitis, chronic cholycestitis, obstructive jaundice, which may be intermittent giving attacks of fever, jaundice and upper abdominal pain-Charcot's triad. Gall bladder empyema from bile duct obstruction is uncommon.

Gallstones are associated with acute and chronic pancreatitis and their presence indicates a higher risk of gall bladder carcinoma although this is still extremely rare.

Management

If causing symptoms, the gall bladder and stones should be removed. It is at this stage that pigment stones are detected and indicate investigation for heamolysis. If the stones are silent they should probably be removed to prevent later trouble. In elderly patients or if surgery is contraindicated, sphincterotomy via ERCP may release the stones. Ursodeoxycholic acid (UDCA) may dissolve translucent (cholesterol) stones in 6-24 months. The stones may recur after treatment.

IV ETIOLOGY AND PATHOGENESIS

1. Stagnation of liver qi:

Emotional stress, worry and anger impede the smooth flow of liver qi. As a result, liver qi stagnates in the liver and gallbladder, and changes into pathogenic heat. The heat steams the bile, resulting in the formation of gallstones.

2. Accumulation of damp-heat

Damp-heat may originate from outside, as a reasonal or epidemic pathogenic factor, or be produced internally, due to impaired spleen and stomach functions caused by improper diet or due to a deficiency state of the spleen which causes its transporting and transforming of water to fail. If, as a result, damp-heat accumulates in the middle-jiao, it will steam the the liver and gallbladder and cause fever and jaundice.

3. Excess of noxious heat

Invasion and accumulation of epidemic noxious heat in the liver and gallbladder impairs yin, blood and the pericardium, leading to high fever, jaundice, mental disorder and bleeding.

V MAIN POINTS OF DIAGNOSIS

1. Acute cholecystitis has an acute onset and persistent pain in the right upper quadrant radiating to the right shoulder accompanied with nausea vomiting and fever. Jaundice may be present in some patients. Physical examination reveals prominent tenderness, rebounding tenderness and muscular tension in the right upper adbomen, sometimes the enlarged gallbladder is palpable.

2. Patients suffering from chronic cholecystitis usually have such chronic symptoms as discomfort in the right upper quadrant, vague pain, abdominal distension, aversion to greasy food, eruction and other dyspeptic manifestation. Physical examination may reveal slight tenderness or no specific signs.

3. Laboratory examination

(1) In the stage of acute attack, leucocytosis, elevated icterus index and hepatic lesion to some extent may be present.

(2) Abdominal X-ray plain film may show positive radioopaqie stone, enlarged gallbladder and calcified opacity. Cholecystography reveals the form of gallbladder and its concentrating function or radio-opaque stone. It is helpful for the diagnosis of chronic cholecystitis.

(3) Duodenal drainage is valuable in detecting the pathogen as well as confirming the diagnosis, giving some hints for treatment. Ultrasonic examination is practical to evaluate the function of gallbladder and suggest the existence of gallstones.

VI DIFFERENTIATION AND TREATMENT
OF COMMON SYNDROMES

1. Damp-heat in the liver and gallbladder (frequently occurring in acute cholecystitis or in acute attack of chronic form)

Main symptoms and signs: alternate spells of fever and chill or fever without chill, pain in the right upper abdomen or right rigs, poor appitite, bitterness in the mouth, even accompanied with nausea and vomiting, constipation, deep-coloured urine, sometimes with jaundice, red tongue with yellow and greasy fur, and taut rapid pulse.

Therapeutic principle: Clearing away pathogenic heat and dampness, soothing the liver and normalizing the function of gallbladder.

Recipe: The combination of Oriental Wormwood Decoction and Decoction of Gentian for Purging Liver-fire with additional ingredients.

Herba Artemisiae Capillaris	30g
Fructus Gardeniae	12g
Radix et Rhizoma Rhei	9g
Radix Scutellariae	15g
Radix Bupleuri	15g
Radix Curcumae	15g
Flos Lonicerae	30g
Fructus Forsythiae	15g
Radix Gentianae	12g
Fructus Aurantii Immaturus	9g
Radix Aucklandiae	9g
Radic Glycyrrhizae	9g

All the above drugs are to be decocted in water for oral administration.

In addition to the above ingredients, 30 grams of gypsum (Gypsum Fibrosum) and 30 grams of isatis root (Radix Isatidis) ought to be employed for the case with high fever; 9 grams of pinellia tuber (Rhizoma Pinelliae) and 9 grams of bamboo shavings (Caulis Bambusae in Taeniam) for the case with nausea and vomiting; 9 grams of chicken's gizzard-skin (Endothelium Corneum Gigeriae Galli) 9 grams of parched hawthorn fruit (Fructus Crataegik) 9 trams of parched medicated leaven (Massa Fermentata Medicinalis) and 9 grams of parched germinated barley (Fructus Hordei Germinatus) fir the case with poor appetite.

2. Stagnation in the liver and gallbladder (frequently occurring in chonic cholecystitis).

Main symptoms and signs: Right-sided hypochondriac pain which sometimes radiates to the right shoulder and back, epigastric distension and fullness, which are aggravated by anger or intake of greasy foods, poor appetite, eruction, nausea, red tongue with thin yellowish fur, and taut pulse.

Therapeutic principle: Soothing the liver and normalizing the function of gallbladder.

Recipe: Modified Major Bupleurum Decoction.

Radix Bupleuri	9g
Radix Scutellariae	9g
Radix Curcumae	15g
Endothelium Corneum Gigeriae Galli	9g
Spora Lygodii	15g
Fructus Aurantii	9g
Radix Aucklandiae	9g
Flos Lonicerae	30g
Fructus Forsythiae	15g
Radix Paeoniae Alba	15g
Radix et Rhizoma Rhei	6g
Radix Glycyrrhizae	6g

All the above drugs are to be decocted in water for oral administration.

Moreover, for the case with poor appetite, 9 grams of parched hawthorn fruit (Fructus Crataegi), 9 grams of parched medicated leaven (Massa Fermentata Medicinalis) and 9 grams of parched germinated barley (Fructus Hordei germinatus) should be administered; for the case with distinct symptoms of spleen deficiency, 9 grams of white atractylodes rhizome (Rhizoma Atractylodis Macrocephalae), 9 grams of dangshen (Radix Codonopsis Pilosulae) and 9 grams of poria (Poria) be administered.

3. Excess of noxious heat

Treatment principal: Clear away heat and toxic materials.

Recipe: Decoction for clearing away heat from gallbladder (Qing Dan

Tang) in this formnla, Radix Bupleuri Regulates liver qi and clears away liver heat; Radix scutellariae, Flos Lonicerae, Herba Taraxaci and Fructus forsythiae clear away heat and eliminate toxic materials; Radix et Rhizoma Rhei and Natrii Sulfas purge excessive heat; Fructus Aurantii Immatures and Rhizoma Pinelliae regulate and harmonize middle jiao; Radix Salviae Miltiorrhizae nourishes blood and eliminates blood stasis.

VII ACUPUNCTURE AND MOXIBUSTION

1. Body acupuncture

A. Main points: Danshu(BL 19), Yanglingquan(GB 34), Taichong(LR 3), Riyue(GB 24), Qimen(LR 14), Zusanli(ST 36).

Danshu, Yanglingquan and Taichong, used together, clear away heat and regulate the flow of liver and gallbladder qi; Riyue and Qimen purge excessive heat in the liver and gallbladder; Zusanli replenishes the spleen and eliminated damp. Reducing method is indicated.

If there is nausea and vomiting, add Zhongwan(RN 12) and Neiguan(PC 6) to harmonize the stomach and arrest the upward adverse flow of qi.

If there is jaundice, add Zhiyang(DU 9) and Xingjian(LR 2) to relieve jaundice.

If there is high fever, add Quchi(LI 11), Dazhui(DU 14) and Hegu(LI 4) to clear away interrior heat.

B. Main points: Tainshu(ST 25) and Zusanli(ST 36)

Supplementary points: Guanyang(RN 14), Pishu(BL 20) and Shangjuxu (ST 37).

Method: All the above points and 1 or 2 of the Supplementary points are punctured each time with moderate stimulation. The meedles are retained for 20 minutes. Moxibustion with moxa stick is applied to Shanque(RN 18) and all the abdominal points. The therapy is given once daily.

C. Main points: Riyue(GB 24), Qimen(LR 14), Danshu(BL 19), Yanglingquan (GB 34), Dannang (EX-LE 6) and Neiguan (PC 6).

Supplementary points: For retention of damp-heat in the interior, Yinlingquan (SP 9) Ququan (LR 8) are added; for calculus of intrahepatic duct,

Taichong(LR 3).

Method: Use the filiform needles to puncture these points with the reducing method.

2. Ear acupuncture

A. Points: Liver Pt, Gallbladder Pt, Stomach Pt, Spleen Pt, Endocrine Pt.

Method: All the points are punctured each time and the eedles are retained for 60 minutes.

B. Prescription: Pt. Liver. Pt. Gallbladder, Pt Sympathetic Nerve, Pt. Shenmen, Pt. Subcortex, Pt. Duodenum, Pt. Stomach and Pt. Large Intestine.

Method: 3-5 points are selected for each treatment. A strong stimulation is given. Retain the needles for 30 minutes. Give the treatment once each day. The auricular-seed-pressing therapy is also applicable.

C. Prescription: Pt. Liver, Pt. Gallbladder, Pt. Sanjiao, Pt. Stomach, Pt. Duodenum, Pt. Esophagus, Pt. Sympathetic Nerve, Pt. Shenmen, Pt. Intertragus (Endocrine) and Pt. Ear Apex.

Method: 3-5 points are selected for each treatment. An electric stimulator is connected to them. Treat with electricity of sparse dense waves for ten minutes ecah time. Give the treatment once a day. The patient should eat two fried eggs in the morning and take magnesium sulfate 15g if he has constipation. During treatment, patient's stools should be sieved and examined for stones.

D. Points: Liver, Gallbladder, Infraantihelix Crus End, Ear Shenmen, Brain, Stomach and Duodenum.

Method: Strong stimulation is used. The needles are retained for 30 minutes. The treatment is given once a day. 3-5 points are used for each treatment, or the seed-embedding method is applicable.

3. Point injection therapy

Points: the same points are selected as in acupuncture therapy.

Drugs: Vitamin B1. Vitamin B_{12} and 5% Chinese angelica solution.

Method: Any one of above drugs can be prescribed and 2 of each of the main and supplementary points are injected with 0.5 millilitre in each. The therapy is given once daily.

VIII QIGONG

A. Cholecystitis

1. Self-treatment by practising qigong

1) Basic maneuvers

It is advisable to practise Six-Character Formula Qigong and Relaxation Qigong.

2) Auxiliary Qigong

(1) Damp-heat type: In is advisable to practise the methods of rubbing the epigastrium and training qi with the word "hu"as well as dredging the spleen and the stomach in Regulating-Spleen Qigong

(2) Qi-stagnation type: It is advisable to practise the methods of rubbing the chest and training qi with the word "xu"as well as soothing the liver and conducting qi in Regulating-Liver Qigong.

2. External qi (Waiqi) therapy

1) Basic maneuvers

(1) First press and knead Pishu (Spleen Shu, BL 20),Ganshu (Liver Shu, BL 18), Danshu(Gallbladder Shu BL 19),Dannang (Gallbladder, EE-LE 6) and Zusanli (Foot Three Li, ST 36), all on the right side of the body.

(2) Apply the flat-palm form, use the vibrating and quivering manipulations to emit qi onto Pishu (Spleen Shu, BL 20), Ganshu (Liver Shu, BL 18) and Danshu (Gallbladder Shu BL 19) for 14 breaths respectively, then emit qi onto the painful area on the front side of the body for 28 breaths.

(3) Apply the flat-palm form, use the pulling and leading manipulations to emit qi onto the gallbladder region on the right front side of the patient for 24 breaths, and conduct qi along the Gall Bladder Channel down to the lower limbs so as to make qi balanced from top to bottom.

2) Auxiliary maneuvers

(1) Qi-stagnation type: Mostly uses the pulling and leading manipulations to conduct qi to the lower limbs.

(2) Apply the flat-palm form, use the pulling and leading manipulations to emit qi onto Zhongwan (Middle Epigastrium, RN 12) and Liangmen (Beam Gate, ST 21) and conduct qi along the Stomach Channel to the lower limbs.

B. Gallstones

1. Self-treatment by Practising Qigong

1) Basic maneuvers

(1) First practise Relaxation Qigong, with stress laid on relaxing the back, waist, chest and hypochondrium. Practise the maneuver repeatedly.

(2) Practise the methods of rubbing the chest and training qi with the word "xu"as well as soothing the liver and conducting qi in Regulating-Liver Qigong.

2) Auxiliary maneuvers

(1) Qi-stagnation type: It is advisable to practise the methods of pushing and conducting to regulate the flow of qi and rubbing the hypochondrium to send down abnormally ascending qi in Sternocostal Qingong as well as the "xu"character formula in Six-Character Formula Qigong.

(2) Dampness-heat type: It is advisable to practise the methods of rubbing the epigastrium and training qi with the work"hu"as well as dredging the spleen and the stomach in Regulating-Spleen Qigong.

2. External qi (Waiqi) therapy

1) Basic maneuvers

(1) First press and knead Pishu (Spleen Shu, BL 20), Weishu (Stomach Shu, BL 21), Ganshu (Liver Shu , BL 18), Danshu (Gallbladder Shu, BL 19), Dannang (Gallbladder, EX-LE 6) and Zusanli(Foot Three Li, ST 36), mainly those on the right side of the body.

(2) Apply the flat-palm form, use the vibrating and quivering manipulations to emit qi onto Pishu (Spleen Shu, BL 20), Weishu (Stomach shu , BL 21), Ganshu (Liver Shu, BL 18) and Danshu (Gallbladder Shu, BL 19) on the right side of the body for 14 breaths respectively, then emit qi onto the painful area on the front side for 28 breaths.

(3) Apply the flat-palm form, use the pulling and quivering manipulations to emit qi onto the gallbladder on the front side of the patient for 24 breaths, and use the pulling and leading manipulations to conduct qi along the Gall Bladder Channel and the Stomach Channel down to the lower limbs.

2) Auxiliary maneuvers

(1) Qi-stagnation type: Chiefly use the pulling and leading manipulations to conduct qi down to the lower limbs so as to make qi balanced from top to bottom.

(2) Damp-heat type: Apply the flat-palm form, use the pulling and leading manipulations to emit qi onto Zhongwan (Middle Epigastrium, RN 12) and Liangmen (Beam Gate, ST 21), and conduct qi along the Stomach Channel down to the lower limbs.

(3) Raise the tongue against the hart palate. The eyes slightly droop. The chest slightly draws in and the back erects. Regulate breathing and concentrate the mind on the back, waist, chest and hypochondrium. Slightly read the word "relax". Practise the maneuver repeatedly (do it over 20 times daily).

IX MASSAGE

Digital-press Ashi points on the back with strong stimulation for 2 to 3 minutes. Then digital-press Dannang(EX-LE6) with strong stimulation for 2 to 3 minutes; pull the vertebrae on the horizontal place of Ashi points on the back with rotating reduction; roll and chafe the both sides of the Bladder meridian for 6 minutes respectively; then press Danshu (BL 19), Ganshu (BL 18) and Geshu (BL 17) for 1 minute respectively; chafe both costal regions; then press and knead Zhangmen(LR 13) and Qimen (LR 14) for 1 minute respectively.

X MEDICATED DIET

Stew pig's trotters to make soup for eating.

Chapter Seven
Ulcerative Colitis

The disease is also termed (Chronic) nonspecific ulcerative colitis. Its etiology is still unknown, but in recent years, is associated with autoimmunity. The pathologic change attacks the rectum, sigmoid colon and descending colon. It is a kind of nonspecific inflammation which primarily involves mucosal layer. Precipitating factors include emotional tonus, psychic trauma and allergy to certain foods. It occurs more frequently in males than in females. In TCM, the disease is categorized as "xie"(diarrhea), "chi bai li"(dysentery), abdominal pain, bloody stool, etc.

I MAIN POINTS OF DIAGNOSIS

1. The disease usually presents in the 20-40 year old group but may occur at any age. First presentation over 65 years is uncommon but carries a greater mortality. At presentation 30% have disease confined to the rectum and 20% have extensive disease.

2. The chief clinical symptoms include diarrhea and abdominal pain. Diarrhea varies in severity. In severe cases it may occur dozens of times a day, accompanied with loose stool, mucous stool or bloody purulent stool and tenesmus. Diarrhea is often perisistent or recurrent and resistant to treatment. In most cases, abdominal pain is localized in the left, middle or lower abdomen, pronounced before defecation and relieved after it. The patients may have fever, anorexia, nausea, loss of weight, anemia, edema, etc. some patients may have erythema nodosum, arthritis, joint pain and other abenteric manifestations.

3. Ulcerative colitis can be divided into three patterns:

A. Chronic recurrent type

The disease may occasionally present as a single short mild episode of diarrhoea which appears to settle rapidly but may at any time relapse.

B. Chronic persistent type

Usually the history is of months or years of general ill health with continuous or intermittent diarrhoea. In these cases the disease is usually restricted to the rectum and descending colon, and then usually termed proctocolitis. General symptoms may be mild or severe. Secondary complications are frequent

C. Fulminant type

Approximately one-fifth of cases present with a severe acute episode of bloody diarrhoea with constitutional symptoms of fever and toxaemia and abodominal distension from toxic megacolon which may proceed to perforation. The first one is more frequent, while the last one, though less frequent, ia in critical condition and its prognosis is poor.

4. Laboratory examination

Routine stool test usually reveals nonspecific changes. Bacterial culture finds no pathogen. Barium enema shows colon spasm and deformity, disordered mucosal folds. In severe case, rigid or dented colon wall, colon stenosis or ulcers can be found. X-ray examination is most helpful in detecting the extent and scope of the disease, but runs a risk in acute phase.

Endoscopy is convenient and the most valuable in the diagnosis, since 95 percent of the patients have rectal involvement. Based on specific morphological changes and biopsy, the diagnosis can be confirmed, and differentiated from colonic or rectal carcinoma, colonic polys or chronic bacillary dysentery.

Sigmoidoscopic appearances: These may be conveniently divided into three groups:

Inactive A granular mucosa with loss of normal vascular pattern.

Active   With pus and blood.

Very active   Pus and blood with contact bleeding at the rim of the sigmoidoscope and visible ulceration.

NB   The rectal mucosa is virtually always abnormal in ulcerative colitis, i. e. it is a distal disease with a variable extension proximately up the large bowel. Histology shows superficial inflammation with chronic inflammatory cells infiltrating the lamina propria, with little involvement of the muscularis mucosa and with reduction of goblet cells.

II OMPLICATIONS

1. General fever, anaemia, weight loss, iatrogenic steroid disease.

2. Colonic loss of protein with hypoalbuminaemia and oedema, loss of electrolytes (sodium and potassium) producing lethargy and contributing to intestinal dilatation. Pseudopolyps are common and possibly predisposing colonic carcinoma.

Carcinoma of the colon is more frequent if the entire colon is involved (total colitis), if the history is prolonged (10% in 10 years), if the first attack was severe, and if the first attack occurred at a young age.

Acute toxic dilatation of the colon with bleeding and perforation still has a high mortality.

3. Non-colonic skin rashes. Erythema nodosum(2%) , (pyoderma) gangrenosum, leg ulcers (2%).

Arthritis (15%)　This usually involves the joints of the hands and feet. Sacroiliitis and ankylosing spondylitis are commoner in patients with ulcerative colitis.

4. Liver disease　Nearly all patients probably have some degree of liver involvement including fatty infiltration, chronic active hepatitis, or pericholangitis, and less commonly sclerosing cholangitis, ascending cholangitis and carcinoma of the bile duct.

These may result from a combination of malnutrition, portal pyaemia, and multiple blood transfusions. Secondary amyloidosis is uncommon but may follow prologed chronic colitis.

5. Ocular iritis and episcleritis occur in about 5% of cases.

6. Venous thrombosis of the legs (5%).

7. Stomatitis (15%).

III DIFFERENTIATION AND TREATMENT OF COMMON SYNDROMES

1. Downward flow of damp-heat (frequently found at the onset or in the duration of the attack)

Main symptoms and signs: Fever, abdominal pain, diarrhea, burning sensation in the anus, or tenesmus, bloody, purulent and mucous stool, red tongue with yellow, thick and greasy fur, and slippery rapid pulse.

Therapeutic principle: Clearing away pathogenic heat and dampness.

Recipe: Decoction of Pueraria, Scutellaria and Coptis with aditional ingredients.

Radix Puerariae	15g
Radix Scutellariae	10g
Rhizoma Coptidis	10g
Flos Lonicerae	30g
Radix Pulsatillae	15g

Semen Plantaginis(wrapped in a piece of cloth before it is decocted)

Radix Aucklandiae	10g
Fructus Aurantii	10g

All the above drugs are to be decocted in water for oral administration.

2. Hyperactivity of the liver and insufficiency of the spleen (often induced by psychic factors)

Main symptoms and signs: Attacks often occurring after emotional tonus and psychic trauma, manifested as abdominal pain before diarrhea, after which the pain is relieved, accompanied with distension and pain in the hypochondrium, epigastric fullness and anorexia, thin and whitish coating of the tongue, and taut thready pulse.

Therapeutic principle: Checking hyperfunction of the liver and strengthening the spleen.

Recipe: Prescription of Importance for Diarrhea with Pain with additional ingredients.

Radix Paeoniae Alba	15g
Rhizoma Atractylodis Macrocephalae	15g
Radix Ledebouriellae	10g
Pericarpium Citri Reticulatae	10g
Radix Bupleuri	10g
Semen Coicis	15g
Semen Dolichoris	12g
Fructus Crataegi	12g

All the above drugs are to be decocted in water for oral administration.

3. Insuffciency of the spleen and stomach (mostly occurring in patients with recurrent attacks)

Main symptoms and signs: Borborygmi, diarrhea with undigested food in the stool, anorexia, stuffiness in the abdomen, lassitude and fatigue, pale tongue with whitish fur, and deep weak pulse.

Therapeutic principle: Reinforcing the spleen and stomach.

Recipe: Modified Powder of Ginseng, Poria and Bighead Astractylodes.

Radix Codonopsis Pilosulae	15g
Semen Nelumbinis	12g
Rhizoma Astractylodis Macrocephalae	12g

Rhizoma Dioscoreae	12g
Semen Dolichoris	9g
Poria	15g
Semen Coicis	15g
Pericarpium Citri Reticulatea	10g
Radix Glycyrrhizae Praeparata	6g

All the above drugs are to be decocted in water for oral administration.

Moreover, 6 grams of aucklandia root (Radix Aucklandiae) and 10 grams of coptis rhizome (Rhizoma Coptidis) ought to be employed for cases with residual heat; 30 grams of halloysite (Halloysitum Rubrum) and 10 grams of nutmeg (Semen Myristicae) for cases with severe diarrhea; 10 grams of chicken's gizzardskin (Endothelium Corneum Gigeriae Galli) for cases with poor appetite.

4. Insufficiency of the spleen-yang and kidney-yang (mostly occurring in the chronic case)

Main symptoms and signs: Diarrhea in the early morning, intolerance of cold, cold limbs, soreness and weakness of the loins, pale and tender tongue with whitish fur, deep thready and weak pulse.

Therapeutic principle: Warming and tonifying the spleen and kidney.

Recipe: Pill of Four Miraculous Drugs with additional ingredients.

Fructus Psoraleae	10g
Semen Myristicae	10g
Fructus Schisandrae	10g
Fructus Evodiae	10g
Radix Aconiti Praepatata	10g
Radix Codonopsis Pilosulae	12g
Rhizoma Atractylodis Macrocephalae	12g
Halloysitum Rubrum	30g
Radix Glycyrrhizae Praeparata	6g

All the above drugs are to be decocted in water for oral administration.

5. Deficiency of the kidney

Main symptoms and signs: Pain below the umbilicus, borborygmi and diarrhoea usually occurring at dawn, abdominal pain relieved after bowel movement and aggravated by cold, abdominal distension sometimes, cold lower extremities. pale tongue with white coating, deep and forceless pulse.

Therapeutic principle: Warm kidney and arrest diarrhea.

Recipe:

Psoralea fruit	9g
Schisandra fruit	9g
Evodia fruit	9g
Nutmeg	9g
Prepared aconite root	9g
Dangshen	15g
Red halloysite	30g
Prepared licorice root	6g

Patent Medicine: Four Divinty Pill (Si Shen Wan). Take 1 pill each time, 3 times a day.

Xie et Liao also classified the affection into three types:

1. Deficiency of the spleen

Deficiency of the spleen fails to keep blood flowing within the vessels, leading to bloody stool. Protracted deficiency of the spleen may attack the kidneys, resulting in deficiency of both the spleen and kidneys. On the other hand, deficiency of the spleen also may cause damp to accumulate in the large intestine.

Main symptoms and signs: Loose and mucopurulent bloody stool, lower abdominal distention or discomfort, sallow complexion, poor appetite, weight loss, pale tongue with deep and small pulse.

Treatment principle: Replenish qi and strengthen the spleen.

Recipe: Guipi Tang (Decoction for Invigorating the Spleen and Nourishing the Heart) and Shen Ling Baizhu San (Powder of Ginseng, Poria and White A-tractylodes); in these prescriptions, Radix Ginseng, Poria, Rhizoma Atractylodis Macrocephalae, Radix Glycyrrhizae, Radix Astragali, Semen Dolichoris Album, Rhizoma Dioscoreae, Semen Nelumbinis and Semen Coicis replenish the spleen and strengthen middle-qi; Radix Angelicae Sinensis nourishes the blood; Radix Aucklandiae and Fructus Amomi regulate qi and harmonize the stomach; other ingredients listed in these prescriptions may be omitted; patients with yang deficiency of both the spleen and kidneys manifested by cold limbs, pallor, lassitude and diarrhea occurring before dawn daiy should receive Sishen Wan (Pill of Four Miraculous Drugs) and Huangtu Tang (Decoction of Baked Yellow Earth); in these formulae, Fructus Psoraleae replenishes fire in the vital gate;

Radix Aconiti Praeparata, Fructus Evodiae and Baked Ginger warm the middle-jiao and expel cold; Semen Myristicae and Fructus Schisandrae are astringents for relieving diarrhea; Radix Rehmanniae and Colla Corii Asini nourish blood; Baked Yellow Earth stops bleeding; and Radix Scutellariae protects the blood from being damaged by drugs that are warm in nature.

2. Accumulation of damp-heat in the middle-jiao

Excessive intake of pungent and greasy food or alcoholic drink causes damp-heat to accumulate in the lower-jiao and damage the intestinal collaterals.

Main symptoms and signs: Loose and mucopurulent bloody stool, lower abdominal pain and tenderness, low-grade fever, thirst with preference for cold drink, reddened tongure wikth yellow, greasy coating and rapid pulse.

Treatment principle: Clear away damp heat.

Recipe: Diyi San (Powder of Radix Sanguisorbae) and Chixiaodou Danggui San (Powder of Phaseolus Seeds and Chinese Angelica Root); in these prescriptions, Radix Sanguisorbae and Radix Rubiae clear away heat from the blood and stop bleeding; Radix Angelicae Sinensis nourishes blood; Radix Scutellariae, Rhizoma Coptidis and Fructus Gardeniae, bitter in taste and cool in nature, cleat away heat and remove damp; Poria and Semen Phaseoli replenish the spleen and remove the damp; if the patient has a greasy tongue coating or fever, add Herb Agastachis and Herba Eupatorii to relieve exterior syndrome and expel damp.

3. Attack of the stagnated liver qi on the spleen

Emotional upset and rage cause liver qi to stagnate, which adversely attacks the spleen, resulting in incoordination between the liver and spleen.

Main symptoms and signs: Diarrhea wisth mucopurulent bloody stool, hypochondriac distension, nausea, irritability, thirst with bitter taste in the mouth, slightly reddened tongue with thin coating and taut pulse.

Treatment principle: Regulate liver qi and strengthen the spleen.

Recipe: Tongxie Yaofang (Prescription of Importance for Diarrhea with Pain); in this prescription, Rhizoma Atractylodis Macrocephalae replenishes the spleen; Radix Paeoniae Alba nourishes blood and harmonizes the liver; pericarpium Citri Reticulatae regulates middle qi; Radix Saposhinkoviae regulates liver qi; if there is marked rectal bleeding, add Flos Sophorae Immatutus, Radix Sanguisorbae, Radix Notoginseng Powder, Rhizoma Blelillae and Herba Agrimoniae.

IV OTHER THERAPIES

1. Enema with herb decoction. 75 to 100 ml concentrated decoction of medicinal herbs is given to the patient once daily. A course includes 30 times and between courses there is an interval of 7 days.

For patients with nonspecific ulcerative colitis who have bloody pus, the following formula is prescribed.

Recipe:

Polygonum multiflorum	15g
Polygonum amplexicaule	15g
Limonium bicolour	30g
Field thistle	30g
Root of garden burnet (baked)	30g
Hyacinth bletilla (tuber)	15g
Rodgersia aesculifolia batal	15g
Copperleaf	30g

Decoction and dosage: All the above herbs make a dose with one dose daily and six to ten doses are prescribed.

For patients with mucus stool, the following formula is prescribed.

Recipe:

Polygonum multiflorum	15g
Polygonum amplexicaule	15g
Hyacinth bletilla	12g
Climbing groundsel	30g
Licorice root	15g
Cortree (bark)	12g
Oldenlandia diffusa (wild.) Roxb	30g
Herba patriniae	30g

Decoction and dosage is the same.

2. Enema with a mixture of the following drugs:

Baiyao	0.4g
Berberine	1g

0. 25% Procain	20ml
0. 9% Nacl sol	60 ml

Dosage. Once daily and a course includes ten times.

3. Enema with sterillized radish juice 100-200 ml, once daily.

4. Herba Portulacae 50g, Radix Pulsatillae 50g and Cortex Phellodendri 50g made into a 100 ml decoction and add 20 ml of 2% procaine, administer enema once daily.

5. Radix Sophorae Flavescentis 30g, Cortex Ailanthi 30g, Radix Pulsatillae 30g, Radix Arnebiae seu Lithospermi 30g and Rhizoma coptidis 10g made into a 200 ml decoction; administer 50-100 ml enema, twice daily.

6. Alumen 9g, Radix et Rhizoma Rhei 6g, Rhizoma Atractylodis 9g, Radix Sophorae Flavescentis 9g and Flos Sophrae 9g made into a 200 ml decoction; administer 50-100 ml enema, daily.

7. Radix Pulsatillae 15g, Cortex Phellodendri 15g, Rhizoma Atractylodis 10g, Rhizoma Polygoni Cuspidati 10g, Radix Angelicae Sinensis 10g, Rhizoma Ligustici 10g, Radix Paeoniae Alba 10g and Fructus Aurantii 10g made into a 200 ml decocton; administer 50-100 ml enema, twice daily.

V ACUPUNCTURE AND MOXIBUSTION

1. Main points: Zhongwan (RN 12), Tianshu (ST 25), Zusanli (ST 36) and Qihai (RN 6) are selected for needling or moxibustion to regulate the function of the stomach and intestines.

Supplementary points:

(1) For deficiency of the spleen, add Pishu (BL 20) and Taibai (SP 3) to strengthen the function of the spleen in transporting and transforming and to stop diarrhea.

(2) For deficiency of the kidneys, add Shenshu (BL 23), Mingmen (DU 4), guanyan (RN 4) and Taixi (KI 3) to reinforce the fire of the vital gate, strengthen the kidneys and promote digestion.

(3) For stagnation of liver qi, add Qimen (LR 14) and Taichong (LR 3) to regulate the flow of qi, remove stagnated liver qi and stop diarrhea.

2. Main points: Pishu (BL 20), and Zusanli (ST 36).

Supplementary points: Add Zhangmen (LR 13), Taibai (SP 3) and Zhongwan (RN 12) for the deficiency of the spleen; add Shenshu (BL 23), Mingmen (DU 4), Guanyuan (RN 4) and Taixi (KI 13) for the deficiency of the kidney.

Method: Apply reinforcing method or moxibustion.

3. Ear acupuncture

Presrcibed points: Large Intestine, Small Intestine, Infraantihelix Crus End, Lung, and Spleen.

Method: Use the seed-embedding method on the both ears alternatively. Change the points once every 3 days.

4. Point injection therapy.

Points: Tianshu(ST 25), Pishu(BL 20), Weishu(BL 21) and Zusanli(ST 36).

Drugs: Vitamin C 500mg.

Method: Each on the above points is injected with 0.5mg of Vitamin C and the therapy is given once daily.

VI MASSAGE

Knead Zhongwan (RN 12), Qihai (RN 6), Guanyuan (RN 4), Tianshu (ST 25) and Jianli (RN 11) for 30 times respectively. Rub Shenque (RN 8), Zhongwan (RN 12) and Dantian to the right for 50 times respectively. Knead Pishu (BL 20) and Shenshu (BL 23) for 30 times respectively. Chafe horizontally the lumbosacral region for 30 times. Press and knead Changqiang(DU 1), Hegu (LI 4), Zusanli (ST 36), Sanyinjiao (SP 6), Weishu (BL 21), Dachangshu (BL 25), Shousanli (LI 10), Mingmen (DU 4) and Taixi (KI 3) for 30 times respectively.

VII QIGONG

1. Place the right hand on Zhongwan (RN 12) and knead from the right to the left for 36 times. Then rub the navel left and right for 36 times.

2. Place the left hand in the underneath with the right hnnd overlapped on

it. Rub the median of the lower abdomen for 36 times. Then the five fingers get closed to knock the lower abdomen slightly for 50 to 100 times.

3. Assume the lying or erect sitting posture. Just before the training practice, drink a small amount of boiled water; loosen the clothes and belt; get rid of all the distracting thoughts and relax the mind. Silently utter phrases generally from 3 Chinese characters to more Chinese characters, but ought not exceed 10 characters at most. The content of the phrases or sentences are usually related to the qigong practice. Meanwhile, coordinate it with respiration exercise; inhale when silently uttering the first word; hold the breath when silently uttering the middle word or words; the more the middle words are, the longer the time of holding breath should be; exhale when silently uttering the final word.

IIX   MEDICATED DIET

1. Make gruel with Chinese yam 15g, euryale seed 9 g, lotus seed 12 g, hyacinth bean 15g , coix seed 15 g, 10 pieces of chinese date, 75g of polished round-grained rice and a right amount of water. Take it twice a day. It is applicable to the patients of the spleen deficiency.

2. Decoct cherokee rose-hip 12g, baked ginger 6 g, nutmeg 6g and schisandra fruit 3 g first and remove the dregs from the decoction. Then add lotus seed 15g, euryale seed 12g, Chinses yam 15g, polished round-grained rice 50g and a right amount of water into it to make gruel. Take the gruel twice a day. It is used to treat the patients of the kidney deficiency.

IX PROGNOSIS

The prognosis is best in those with disease confined to the rectum (ulcerative proctitis): only about 10% of these develop complications. About 70% of all cases remit with medical treatment in the first attack, 15% improve, and 15% come to surgery or die. The excess mortality is chiefly within the first year of presentation. In 10 years 30% have extensive disease, 15% need surgery, and 10% have colonic disease. Young patients do better than old patients, and subtotal colitis is less severe than total colitis in terms of both general health and the risk of colonic carcinoma. Surgery is therefore indicated early in patients who are older and have total colitis. The mortality from total colectomy when performed as a 'cold' procedure is 2-4% (inseverely ill acute cases including toxic dilatation the mortality may be as high as 30-40%). However, 20% of these patients require further surgery usually to refashion the stoma or less commonly to divide obstructing adhesions. Impotence and loss of micturition control are serious complications of surgery.

Chapter Eight
Constipation

I DIFFERENTIATION AND TREATMENT
OF COMMON SYNDROME

1. Heat constipation type

Main symptoms and signs: Constipation, difficult defecation, one defecation every 3 to 5 days or even longer, fever, thirst, foul breath, scanty dark urine, anorexia. Yellow and dry tongue coating, slippery, replete and forceful pulse.

Therapeutic principle: Clear away the heat and moisten the intestines to relieve constipation.

Recipe:

Rhubarb   9g

Hemp seed	30g
Bitter apricot kernel	12g
White peony root	15g
Immature bitter orange	12g
Magnolia bark	12g
Dried rehmannia root	30g
Scrophularia root	30g
Ophiopogon root	15g

All the above drugs are decocted in water for oral odministration.

Patent Medicine: Hemp Seed Pill (Maziren Wan). Take 9g each time, twice a day.

2. Qi constipation type

Main symptoms and signs: Constipation, fullness and distending pain in the abdomen and hypochodriac regions, frequent belching, loss of appetite. Thin and greasy tongue coating, wiry pulse.

Therapeutic principle: Smoothen qi and remove stagnation.

Recipe:

Aucklandia root	15g
Lindera root	15g
Eagle wood	9g
Rhubarb root	9g
Areca seed	15g
Immature bitter orange	15g

All the above drugs are decocted in water for oral adminstration.

Patent medicine: Immature Bitter Orange Stagnation-removing Pill (Zhishi Daozhi Wan). Take 9g each time, twice a day.

3. Deficient constipation type

Main symptoms and signs: Constipation, sweat and short breath during the defecation, pale and lustreless complexion, dizziness, blurred vision, pale lips and nails, palpitation, lassitude. Pale tongue with thin coating, thready and weak pulse.

Therapeutic principle: Tonify qi and nourish blood, moisten the intestines and relieve constipation.

Recipe:

Astragalus root	30g
Hemp seed	30g
Honey	30g
Tangerine peel	15g
Dried rehmannia root	30g
Chinese angelica root	30g
Peach kernel	9g
Bitter orange	9g

All the above drugs are decocted in water for administration

Patent medicine: five Kernels Pill(Wu RN Wan). Take 9g each time, 3 time a day.

II ACUPUNCTURE AND MOXIBUSTION

1. Body acupuncture

Main points: Dachangshu (BL 25), Tianshu (ST 25), Zhigou (SJ 6), and Zhaohai(KI 16).

Supplementary points: Add Quchi (LI11) and Hegu (LI4) for heat constipation; Zhongwan (RN 12) and Taichong (LR 3) for constipation due to stagnation of qi; Pishu (BL 20), Weishu (BL 21) and Zusanli (ST 36)for deficiency of qi and blood.

Method: Apply the filiform needles with sedation for heat constipation and constipation due to stagnation of qi, and with tonification for deficient constipation.

2. Ear acupuncture

Prescribed points: Lower Rectum, Large Intestine, and Brain.

Method: Twist the needles with moderate or strong stimulation and retain the needles for 20-30 minutes.

III. MASSAGE

Knead Tianshu (ST 25), Guanyuan(RN 4), Shenshu (BL 23) Zhishi (BL 52) and Changqiang (GV 1) for 30 times respectively. Rub the lower abdomen clockwise for 50 times. Press and knead Pishu (BL 20), Weishu (BL 21), Dachangshu (BL 25), Hegu (LI4), Shousanli (LI 10), Zusanli (ST 36), Taichong (LR 3), Zhigou (SJ 6) and Zhangmen (LR 13) for 30 times respectively. Pat the shank for 10 times. Grasp Chengshan (BL 57) for 10 times and chafe Yaoyan (EX-B7) for 30 times.

IV MEDICATED DIET

1. Infuse 2 to 3 whole pieces of boat-fruited sterculia seed and proper amount of white sugar with boiling water to drink at any time as tea.

2. Infuse 3 g of senna leaf with boiling water to drink as tea, 3 times a day.

3. Take honey alone or add it into boiling water or milk to drink at any time.

4. Take water chestnut 30 to 60 g each time, at any time.

V QIGONG

1. Assume the sitting posture or the supine posture. Relax the whole body, breathe naturally. Raise the tongue tip against the hard palate, and concentrate the mind on the area of the navel. With the navel as the center, activate the abdominal muscles in inhalation. Conduct qi with the mind to rotate upward and leftward from the lower portion of the right abdomen, silently reading " The white tiger hides in the east"; in exhalation, conduct qi to rotate from above to below to the right from the upper portion of the left abdomen, silently reading "The blue dragon shelters in the west". Circulate for a circle in this way. With the navel as the center, rotate from small circles to large ones clockwise for 36 circles altogether up to sides of the abdomen.

2. In exhalation, push with the respective 4 fingers of the two hands or the whole palms the median line of the abdomen from the xiphoid process to the sym-

physis pubis for 36 times and then push obliquely downwards from the xiphoid process to the bilateral sides for 36 times. The mind is concentrated on the pushing and rubbing sensation beneath the hands.

3. Place the right hand on Zhongwan (RN 12) and rub from the right to the left for 36 times. Then rub and knead the navel area left and right for 36 times.

Chapter Nine
Diarrhea

Diarrhea is defined as an increase in the frequency, fluidity and volume of bowel movements. Normal bowel function varies from individual to individual, and the definition of diarrhea must take this variation into account. Factors influencing stool consistency are poorly understood; water content is not the sole determinant, thus, the definition of diarrhea in a clinical sense is an increase in frequency or increased fluidity of bowel movements in a given individual. In pathophysiologic terms, diarrhea results from the passage of stools containing excess water, i. e. from malabsorption or secretion of water.

Most diarrheal states are self-limited and pose no special diagnostic problem. They are often due to dietary indiscretions or mild gastrointestinal infections. The following list of the causes of diarrhea is indicative of the extensive diagnostic eveluation that may be required in patients with unexplained, profound or chronic diarrhea.

The many causes for diarrhea may be briefly outlined as follows:

1. Functional disorders including adaptive colitis, allerty to ingested food and drugs, defective gastric or pancreatic digestion, defective absorption, vitamin deficiencies and abuse of cathartic.

2. Generalized disorder or disease affecting the intestine, including uremia, Graves' disease, Addison's disease, cardiac decompensation, portal hypertension, neurologic disease and poisoning with heavy metals.

3. Intrinsic disease of the intestine, due to:

A. Specific biral, bacterial and fungal infection, protozoan, or metazoan parasites;

B. Alterations in intestinal flora, antimicrobial therapy, fistula, blind loops, or small intestinal stasis;

C. Nonspecific inflammatory disease such as regional enteritis or ulcerative colitis;

D. Benign or malignant tumors and other causes of partial intestinal obstruction.

In traditional Chinese medicine, diarrhea is thought to be caused by inability of the body to regulate water, resulting in stasis of dampness in the stomach and intestine, or in the spleen. In diarrhea, kidney, large intestine and liver are often involved.

I. MAIN SYMPTOMS AND SIGNS

With excess fecal water:

Osmotic diarrhea-Excess water-soluble molecules in the bowel lumen cause osmotic retention of intraluminal water.

Secretory diarrhea-Excessive active ion secretion by the mucosal cells of the intestine.

Deletion or interference with normal ion absorption-This is usually a congenital problem.

Exudative disease-Abnormal mucosal permeability with intestinal loss of serum proteins, blood, mucus pus.

Impaired contact between intestinal chyme and absorbing surface-Rapid transit, short bowel syndromes.

Without excess fecal water-frequent, small, painful evacuations are usually a result of disease of the left colon or rectum.

II DIFFERENTIATION AND
TREATMENT OF COMMON SYNDROMES

In traditional Chinese medicine, diarrhea is divided into five types.

1. Chang pi type: Chang pi is an acute intestinal infection commonly seen in summer and autumn, and characterized by watery diarrhea, cramp of the gas-

trocnemius muscles of the leg due to excessive loss of water from severe vomiting and diarrhea, thirst, dark urine and profuse sweating, mucoid glossy coating of the tongue. The formula for this type is Qin Sao Wei Lin Tang Jia Jian.

Recipe:

Skullcap	10g
Root of herbaceous peony	30g
Chinese atractylodes	15g
Bark of official magnolia	10g
Dried old orange peel	12g
Pinellia	10g
Tuckahoe	30g
Umbellate pore	12g
Oriental water plantain	12g
Asiatic plantain	30g
Wrinkled leaven	12g
Leaf of purple perilla	12g

All the above drugs are decocted in water for oral administration.

Decoction and dosage: All the above herbs make a dose and six to ten doses are prescribed with one dose daily. Each dose is simmered twice and then the broth of each mixed, half of the mixed broth each time, twice a day.

2. Heat type: Heat type diarrhea is due to the invasion of a pathogenic heat factor into the large intestine. The chief symptoms are diarrhea with very foul mucoid stools, borborygmus, abdominal pains, burning sensation of the anus, scanty dark urine, thirst, tenesmus, yellow coating of the tongue, rapid pulse. The treatment is to dissipate heat with Ge Gen Qin Lian Tang Jia Jian.

Recipe:

Root of kudzuvine	15g
Skullcap	10g
Chinese goldthread	10g
Chinese pulsatilla	20g
Corktree	12g
Ash bark	12g
Purslane	30g
Fruit of hawthorn	30g

Betal nut   15g

All the above drugs are decocted in water for oral odministration. Decoction and dosage is the smae.

3. Food type: Food type diarrhea is caused by improper or contaminated diets, clinically it is manifested as belching, regurgitation of acid, poor appetite, distress of the chest and epigastrium, abdominal pain followed and relieved by diarrhea, thick coating of the tongue, etc. The treatment is intended to relieve food accumulation with Bao He wan Jia Jian.

Recipe:

Fruit of hawthorn	30g
Medicated leaven	30g
Malt	30g
Weeping forsythia	15g
Chinese radish seed	18g
Dried old orange peel	12g
Pinellia	12g
Wrinkled leaven	12g
Membrane of chincken gizzard	10g
Rhubarb	6g

Decoction and dosage is the same.

4. The type of deficiency of the spleen-yang. The pathologic manifestations cf the decline of splenic functions together with the cold syndrome. The main symptoms are distension, chilliness and pain of epigastrium, anorexia, loose stools or chronic diarrhea or chronic dysentery, cold limbs, pale tongue with whitish coating, empty and slow pulse, etc. The treatment is to warm and strengthen the spleen with Shen Lin Bai Su San Jia Jian.

Recipe:

Dangshen	12g
Large-headed atractylodes (baked)	30g
Chinese atractylodes	15g
Chinese yam rhizome	30g
Bean of white hyacinth dolichos	30g
Semen coicis	10g
Coix seed	30g

Hibdu lotus	12g
Dried old orange peel	12g
Pinellia	12g
Tuckahoe	30g
Fruit of hawthorn	30g
Medicated leaven	30g
Malt	30g
Monkshood (root)	10g
Wrinkled leaven	12g

Decoction and dosage is the same.

5. The type of deficiency of kidney-yang. The patients with this type of diarrhea always complain of diarrhea before dawn with clilliness of the abdomen, cold limbs, impaired appetite, chill and pain of the waist and knees, abdominal pain which can be relieved by discharge of the feces, pale tongue, small formicant pulse, etc. The treatment is to invigorate the kidney-yang with Shi Sheng Wan Jia Jian.

Recipe:

Nutmeg	12g
Malaytea scurfpea	12g
Fruit of Chinese Magnolia vine	12g
Evodia fruit	10g
Chinese yam rhizome	30g
Chinese atractylodes	15g
Large-headed atractylodes	30g
Coix seed	30g
Bean of white hyacinth dolichos	30g
Bark of Chinese cassia tree	2g
Dried ginger	10g
Licorice root	6g

Decoction and dosage is the asme.

III ACUPUNCTURE AND MOXIBUSTION

Main points: Tianshu(ST 25), Dachangshu(BL 25) and Zusanli(ST 36).

Supplementary points: Zhongwan(RN 12) for cold-damp syndrome; Neiting(ST 44), Yinlingquan(ST 9) and Hegu(LI 4) for damp-heat syndrome; Pishu(BL 20), Zhangmen(LR 13), Taibai(SP 3) and Zhongwan(RN 12) for deficiency of the yang and spleen.

Method: All the main points are punctured together with the auxiliary ones which are selected according to the symptoms. The puncture is moderate and the needles are retained for 20 minutes. The therapy is given once daily. Moxibustion is applied to Baihui(DU 20) to raise qi of the spleen and stomach.

IV CUTTING THERAPY

Points for cutting: Pishu(BL 20) and Shenshu(BL 23).

Method: Carefully sterilize the skin of the points before infiltration anesthesia with 1 ml novocain. A longitudinal incision is conducted on the point and a little subcutaneous fatty tissue is removed. Then the cut is sutured and dressed. The stitch is removed a week later and the second therapy is given 2 or 3 weeks afterwards.

Chapter Ten
Spasm of Diaphragm

I DIFFERENTIATION AND TREATMENT OF COMMON SYNDROMES

1. Cold accumulation in the stomach

Main symptoms and signs: Deep, slow and forceful hiccup, aggravated by cold and relieved by warmth, discomfort in the diaphragm and epigastrium, preference for hot drinks, no thirst. White tongue coating, delayed pulse.

Therapeutic principle: Warm the centre and disperse the cold, suppress the reversely-flowing qi and stop hiccup.

Recipe:

Cloves	9g
Kaki calyx	9g
Galangal rhizome	6g
Citron fruit	9g
Magnolia bark	9g
Tangerine peel	9g
Prepared licorice root	6g

All the above drugs are decocted in water for oral administration

2. Qi stagnation and phlegm obstruction

Main symptoms and signs: Hiccup with phlegm obstruction, difficulty in respiration, fullness and distension in the epigastrium and hypochondria, borborygmus, flatus, or accompanied by nausea and belching, dizziness, blurred vision, epigastric stuffiness, poor appetite. Thin and greasy tongue coating, wiry and slippery pulse.

Therapeutic principle: Regulate qi and dissipate phlegm, suppress the reversely-flowing qi and stop hiccup.

Recipe:

Inula flower	9g
Red ochre	15g
Pinellia tuber	9g

Fresh ginger	6g
Bamboo shavings	9g
Tangerine peel	9g
Poria	12g

All the above drugs are decocted in water for oral administration.

3. Yang deficiency of the spleen and kidney

Main symptoms and signs: Low and long hiccup, shortness of breath, watery vomiting, discomfort in the abdomen, preference for warmth and pressure, lustreless complexion, poor appetite, lassitude. Pale tongue with thin and white coating, thready and weak pulse.

Therapeutic principle: Warm and tonify the spleen and kidney, harmonize the stomach and suppress the reversely-flowing qi.

Recipe :

Prepared aconite root	9g
Dried ginger	6g
Dangshen	12g
White atractylodes rhizome	12g
Cloves	9g
Nutmeg	6g
Chinese yam	15g
Evodia fruit	6g
Prepared licorice root	6g

All the above drugs are decocted in water for oral administration.

II SIMPLE AND CONVENIENT RECIPE

1. Collect loquat leaf 60g and brush off the downs. Add 600 ml water and decoct it into 150 ml decoction to drink.

2. Smash fresh ginger 30g to get juice and throw the dregs; then mix the juice wsith honey 30g and take it all at once.

3. Decoct pumpkin calyx 4 pieces and drink the decoction continuously for 3 to 4 times.

III ACUPUNCTURE AND MOXIBUSTION

1. Body acupuncture

Main points: Neiguan (PC6), and Geshu (BL17).

Supplementary points: Add Zusanli (ST 36) and Zhongwan (RN 12) for fullness and distension in the epigastrium; add Guanyuan (RN 4) for lingering hiccup due to weak body constitution.

Method: The filiform needles are used with sedation and retained for 20 minutes. Moxibustion can be used on Guanyuan (RN 4).

2. Ear acupuncture

Prescribed points: Diaphragm, Stomach, Ear-Shenmen, Spleen, Infraantihelix Crus End.

Method: The filiform needles are punctured with medium stimulation and retained for 20 minutes. The intradermal needle or seed-embedding method can be applicable. In the seizure of hiccup, the patient is asked to press it himself till hiccup disappears.

3. Cupping therapy

Prescribed points: Danzhong (RN 17), Zhongwan (RN 12), Juque (RN 14), Weishu (BL 21), Geshu (BL 17), and Pishu (BL 20).

Method: Two points are chosen each time and the cups are retained for 15 minutes.

IV MASSAGE

Press and knead Geshu (BL17) and Weishu (BL21) for 2 to 3 minutes respectively; apply the chafe method along the Bladder Meridian of Foot-Taiyang downwards from Xinshu (BL15) to Weishu (BL21) till there is a warm sensation in the local area. Press and knead Danzhong (RN17) and Zhongwan (RN12) for 2 to 3 minutes respectively; then apply the divergent moving method with two hands outwards from Zhongting (RN16) to the two hypochondria; finally press Zusanli (ST36), Taichong (LR3) and Neiting (ST44) for 2 minutes respectively.

Chapter Eleven
Infantile Anorexia

I DIFFERENTIATION AND TREATMENT OF COMMON SYNDROME

1. Qi dificiency in the spleen and stomach

Main symptoms and signs: Prolonged poor appitite, stools with undigested food, pale complexion, mental fatigue, spontaneous perspiration. Pale tongue with thin and white coating, thready pulse. red superficial venule of the index finger.

Therapeutic principle: Invigorate the spleen, replenish qi and harmonize the stomach.

Recipe:

Aucklandia root	6g
Amomum fruit	3g
Chinese yam	12g
Hyacinth·bean	9g
Caryophyllaceous ginseng	12g
White atractylodes rhizome	9g
Poria	9g
Prepared licorice	3g

All the above drugs are decocted in water for oral administration

Patent medicine: Aucklandia, Amomum and Six Nobles Pill (Xiangsha Liujunzi Wan). Take 3 g each time, three times a day.

2. Impairment by improper diet

Main symptoms and signs: Food refusal due to improper feeding, sour and fetid stool or constipation, abdominal distention or pain, nausea, vomiting, restlessness. Red tongue with thick and greasy coating, slippery pulse, purple and stagnant superficial venule of the index finger.

Therapeutic principle: Promote the flow of qi to remove stagnated food.

Recipe:

Round cardamon seed	6g

Magnolia bark	6g
Shell of areca nut	9g
Radish seed	6g
Chinken's gizzard-skin	9g
Germinated barley	9g
Hawthorn fruit	12g
Forsythia fruit	9g

All the above drugs are decocted in water for oral administration

Patent medicine: Infantile Stagnated-Food-Removing Pill (Xiaoer Xiaoji Wan). Take 5 pills for 1-3 months old, 10 pills for 3-6 months, 20 pills for 6-12 months, 30 pills for 1-2 years, 50 pills for 2-6 years each time (320 pills are equal to 1g), twice a day.

II SIMPLE AND CONVENIENT RECIPE

Grind poria into fine powder. Take 6g with warm boiled water each time, twice a day.

III ACUPUNCTURE AND MOXIBUSTION

Main points: Zhongwan (RN12), Zhangmen (LR13), Pishu (BL20), Weishu (BL21), and Zusanli (ST36).

Supplementary points: Add Sifeng (EX-UE10) for impairment by improper diet.

Method: The filiform needles are applied with tonification once a day. Sifeng (EX-UE10) is pricked with a three-edged needle to cause discharge of a little bit of yellowish fluid by means of sqeezing.

IV MASSAGE

Put some medium on the child's back. Press and knead lightly along the middle of spine from top to bottom for 3 times. Lift and grasp the skin heavily and simultaneously with the palmar side of the thumb which is held out against

the skin, index and middle fingers, and grasp forword with two hands alternatively from the end of coccyx to Dazhui (DU 14). Press and knead Shenshu
(BL23) for 5 times.

V MEDICATED DIET

1. Grind 6g pieces of chicken's gizzard-skin, 3g of tangerine peel and 2g of
amomum fruit into powder; make gruel with 30g of polished round-grained rice
and add the powder after the gruelis done. Take it as refreshment.

2. Have the crust of cooked millet baked dry and ground into powder. Take
it with the water of brown sugar.

VI NURSING

Feeding should be proper to avoid developing into food retention. Diet ought
to be various and well arranged. Take less sugar and no fried food.

Chapter Twelve
Epidemic Parotitis

I. DIFFERENTIATION AND TREATMENT
OF COMMON SYNDROME

1. Epidemic toxicity in the exterior

Main symptoms and signs: Aversion to cold, fever, headache, mild cough,
pain of the parotid region below the ear, difficulty in chewing, swelling and pain
of the parotid glands on one or both sides without definite margins. Light red
tongue with thin and white coating, superficial and rapid pulse.

Therapeutic principle: Dispel the wind and clear away the heat scatter the
accumulation and relieve the swelling.

Recipe:

Honeysuckle flower   15g

Forsythia fruit	9g
Isatis root	9g
Prunella spike	9g
Platycodon root	9g
Peppermint(Decoct later)	6g
Arctium fruit	6g
Scutellaria root	9g
Licorice root	3g

All the above drugs are decocted in water for oral administration

2. Accumulation of heat and toxicity

Main symptoms and signs: High fever, headache, restlessness, thirst, poor appetite, or vomiting, general lassitude, swelling of the parotid glands with burning pain, red and swollen throat, difficulty in chewing and swallowing, dry stools, scanty and dark urine. Red tongue with thin, greasy and yellow coating, slippery and rapid pulse.

Therapeutic principle: Clear away the heat and relieve the toxicidty, soften the hardness and remove the swelling.

Recipe:

Scutellaria root	9g
Scrophularia root	9g
Arctium fruit	9g
Isatis root	15g
Batryticated silkworm	9g
Platycodon root	9g
Peppermint(Decoct later)	6g
Prunella spike	15g
Dandelion herb	9g
Gypsum	30g
Anemarrhena rhizome	15g

All the above drugs are decocted in water for oral administration

II ACUPUNCTURE AND MOXIBUSTION

1. Body acupuncture

Main points: Shuaigu (GB8), Yifeng (SJ17), Jiache (ST6), and Hegu (LI4).

Supplementary points: Add Quchi (LI11) and Waiguan (SJ5) for severe cases; add Taichong (LR3) and Ququan (LR8) for swelling of the testis.

Method: Use the filiform needles to puncture the points with the reducing method. Puncture Shuaigu (GB8) 1. 5 inches deep subcutaneously toward the ear apex, making the needling sensation to reach the diseased part. Retain the needles for 30 minutes. Give the treatment once a day.

2. Ear acupuncture

Prescribed points: Parotid Gland, Cheek, and Brain.

Method: Apply a strong stimulation. Retain the needles for 20 minutes. Give the treatment once each day. Or use the auricular seed-embedding method.

Chapter Thirteen
Bacillary Dysentery

Bacillary dysentery is an infectious disease of the intestinal tract causcd by Shigella. It commonly occurs in summer and autumn. The disease is transmitted by means of contact with the contaminated food, water and tableware. The major pathological change is the purulent inflammation of the colonic mucosa. Clinically, fever, abdominal pain, diarrhea, tenesmus and bloody purulent stools are major manifestations. In TCM, this desease belongs to the category of "li ji" (dysentery).

I MAIN POINTS OF DIAGNOSIS

Bacillary dysentery can be divided into acute and chronic types according to the clinical features and courses.

1. Acute bacillary dysentery

(1) In epidemic seasons, the history of eating contaminated food and close contact with dysentery is helpful to diagnosis.

(2) The onset is often abrupt. The patients complain of chill sensation, fever, pantalgia, abdominal cramps and diarrhea. The abdominal pain is mainly around the umbilicus or at the left lower quadrant. The bowel movements may be more than ten times a day. Initially , the stools are soft and yellow in colour, and subsequently are mucopurulent and bloody, accompanied with tenesmus. A few patients, because of old age, general asthenia or having chronic disease, may have trance or cama. The prognosis of patient manifested as severe toxemia or infectious shock is very poor.

(3) Laboratory findings: White blood cell counts are increased with a shift to the left in the differential count. Microscopic examination of the stool reveals a great number of erythrocytes, leukocytes and pus cells and a few macrophages. Stool culture can confirm the diagnosis and identify the causing organisms.

2. Chronic bacillary dysentery

(1) Having a past history of acute bacillary dysentery or a history of chronic persistent course due to the inadequate treatment for acute bacillary dysentery.

(2) Having recurrent or persistent abdominal pain, accompanied eith diarrhea or alternation of diarrhea and constipation. Intermittent appearance of mucopurulent and blood-stained stools. Patients of long duration of the disease may appear weak, emaciated and malnourished.

(3) Definite diagnosis can be made when stool culture is positive. Sigmoidoscopy is reserved for the cases difficult to diagnose.

II DIFFERENTIATION AND
TREATMENT OF COMMON SYNDROMES

1. Dysentery due to damp-heat pathogen (Occuring in acute bacillary dysentery)

Main symptoms and signs: Abdominal pain, diarrhea with bloody mucous stool which is moved several times or more than ten times a day with a small amount each time, tenesmus, burning sensation at the anus, scanty deep-coloured urine, or accompanied with chill and fever, yellow and greasy coating of the tongue, slippery and rapid pulse.

Therapeutic principle: Clearing away heat and eliminating dampness and regulating qi to remove stagnancy.

Recipe: Modified Peony Decoction.

Radix Paeoniae Alba	20g
Rhizoma Coptidis	10g
Radix Scutellariae	10g
Flos Lonicerae	30g
Herba Portulacae	30g
Radix et Rhizoma Rhei	6g
Redix Aucklandiae	6g
Semen Arcae	10g
Fructus Aurantii	10g
Radix Glycyrrhizae	6g

All the above drugs are to be decocted in water for oral administration.

For the case with the onset of chill and fever, 15 grams of pueraria root (Rhizoma Puerariae) Is usually added.

2. Fulminant dysentery (Mostly occuring in toxic bacillary dysentery)

Main symptoms and signs: Sudden onset, violent attack, purulent and bloody stools, or bloody stools, high fever, restlessness or even coma or convulsion in serious cases, red tongue or deep-red tongue with yellow greasy fur and rapid pulse.

Therapeutic principle: Removing heat and toxic materials and cooling the blood.

Recipe: Modified Pulsatilla Decoction.

Radix Pulsatillae	30g
Cortex Fraxini	15g
Rhizoma Coptidis	10g
Cortex Phellodendri	10g
Flos Lonicerae	30g
Fructus Forsythiae	15g
Cortex Moutan Radicis	10g
Radix Paeoniae Rubra	10g
Radix Sanguisorbae	15g

Radix Puerariae   15g

All the above drugs are to be decocted in water for oral administration.

If there appears coma, convulsion or toxic shock, Bezoar Sedative Bolus, Purple Snowy Powder and the like may be added. Meanwhile, the treatment of TCM should be given in combination with that of Western medicine.

3. Recurrent dysentery (mostly found in chronic bacillary dysentery)

Main symptoms and signs: Chronic dysentery with frequent relapse, and slow recovery, abdominal pain and tenesmus during the attack, dark-coloured mucous stools, fatigue and weakness, pale tongae with greasy fur, deep and weak pluse.

Therapeutic principle: Invigorating the spleen, replenishing qi, removing heat and eliminating dampness.

Recipe: Modified Decoction of Four Noble Drugs.

Radix Codonopsis Pilosulae	15g
Rhizoma Atractylodis Macrocephalae	10g
Poria	15g
Radix Aucklandiae	10g
Rhizoma Coptidis	10g
Radix Pulsatillae	20g
Radix Sanguisorbae	15g
Radix Glycyrrhizae Praeparata	6g

All the above drugs are to be decocted in water for oral administration.

If yin-blood is injured with symptoms of irritability, thirst, red tongue with little fur, fine and rapid pulse, 15 grams of dried rehmannia root (Radix Rehmanniae), 12 grams jof white peony root (Radix Paeoniae Alba) and 12 grams of black plum (Fructus Mume) are to be added.

If the case is ascribed to dysentery of deficiency-cold type with symptoms of watery and purulent stools, abdominal pain with preference for warmth and pressure, cold extremities, loss of appetite, listlessness, pale tongue with whitish fur, deep and fine pulse, it is preferable to employ Modified Decoction for Nourishing the Viscera, including: dangshen(Radix Codonopsis Pilosulae) 12g, white atractylodes rhizome(Rhzoma Atractylodis Macrocephalae) 10g, baked ginger (Rhizoma Zingiberis) 10g, cinnamon bark (Cortex Cinnamomi) 6g, nutmeg (Semen Myristicae) 10g, chebula fruit (Fructus Chebulae) 15g, aucklandia root

(Radix Aucklandiae) 6g, red halloysite (Halloysitum Rubrum) 12g, pomegranate rind (Pericarpium Granati) 15g, prepared licorice root (Radix Glycyrrhizae Praeparata) 6g. All the above ingredients are to be decocted in water for oral administration.

Chapter Fourteen
Carcinoma of Esophagus

Carcinoma of the esophagus (EC) is the most frequently encountered malignant tumors in China. According to recent investigations, it is the most prevalent neoplasm of the upper alimentary tract in some districts of China. The mortality rate of malignant tumors is around 700,000 per year, 158,000 of which belong to EC. The age of onset is over 40 in most cases, two thirds occuring between the ages of 50 to 70. The disease is eight times more common among men than among women.

The cause of EC is complicated. Most EC is the combined result of many factors. It is assumed that smoking, drinking, eating hot and coarse food, fermented Chinese sauerkraut, ingestion of carcinogenic chemicals, malnutrition, poor hygienic conditions in oral cavity, chronic esophagitis, hereditory factors or immunological dysfunction are relevant to the etiology of esophageal carcinoma.

50% of EC are in the middle third of the esophagus, 30% in the distal third and the remaining 20% in the upper third. 90% of them appear in the squamous carcinoma, the others are adenocarcinoma, adenospino-carcinoma and undifferentiated carcinoma. It also extends itself by direct local invasion into the wall of esophagus. Metastasis through hematogenous dissemination of the entire body usually occurs in the advanced stage.

I GENERAL INTRODUCTION TO THE PATHOGENESIS

This disease, ascribed to the general debility and deficiency of both qi and blood in the aged, is often induced by emotional stimuli or improper diet, which causes the scorching of pathogenic heat in the stomach depletion of body fluid, choking sensation on swallowing and the subsequent blockage of the esophagus.

The lower orifice is usually first obstructed, manifesting as dry stool of sheep-faece-shape. Then qi will go upwards due to the blockage, leading to profuse and thick fluid in the mouth and stabbing pain in the chest and back and finally the formation of the critical disease.

II MAIN SYMPTOMS AND SIGNS

Progressive dysphagia is the most prominent symptom of the disease which is usually associated with frequent vomiting of thick fluid dry stool and painful chest and diaphragm. At the advanced stage, enlarged lymph nodes, severe weight loss, difficult and unsmooth swallowing of liquid meal may appear as a result of the disease invading channels and collaterals.

Stagnation of qi in the middle-jiao caused by anxiety and worry often lead to the blockage of the ascending and descending movement of qi. At a result, inability of the stomach qi in descending forces the turbid-qi going upward adversely and gives rise to the obstruction in the chest. Excessive foggy fluid in the chest that fails to be distributed will be transformed into phlegm or thick fluid. For this reason, swallowing becomes difficult and frequent vomiting of fluid presents. In most cases, the pulse is moderate and slippery, and the tongue coating is whitish and thick, showing that there is stagnation of qi and accumulation of dampness.

Pain in the hypochondrium is brought up by the stagnation of the spleen qi leading to the depression of liver and blockage of qi in the gallbladder channels while forceful and taut pulse and red tongue are caused by the stagnation of fire resulting from the stagnant qi.

The liver relies on the spleen to aid the heart fire. Stagnation of qi in the middle-jiao and sinking of the spleen qi will obstruct the way of the liver qi to go upward, leading to debility of the depressed liver to dredge the actions of orifices and the ensuing difficult defecation. Furthermore, spleen dampness, adverse flow of the stomach qi depression of the lung and exuberance of phlegm may all disturb the production of body fluid and lead to the shortage of fluid in the intestine. So defecation becomes difficult and the feces is as dry as that of a sheep. In most cases of this type, the tongue is dark, blue and purple, the coating is thick, greasy or smooth, indicating that the disease is in the advanced stage.

Determination of the deficiency fo excess of syndromes according to the symptoms and signs:

Vomiting of profuse thick fluid indicates excess of dampness and deficiency of the spleen.

Nausea, vomiting and epigastric fullness and distension suggest inability of the stomach qi to descend and upward invasion of the liver qi.

Chest distension and cough show the upflaring of the liver fire due to rage impairing the liver.

Frequent urination and urinary incontinence are signs of original deficiency of the kidney and fire derived from emotional injury.

Determination of the deficiency or excess of syndromes according to complexion and pulse:

Red lustrous complexion, large and forceful pulse, vomiting and nausea right after eating with sour and fetid smell indicete an excess syndrome due to heat.

Blue pallor or pallor yellowish and lustreless complexion or withered face, weak and hollow pulse, vomiting in the evening containing the food taken in the morning or cold watery vomitus without sour or fetid smell suggest a deficiency syndrome due to cold.

Tense and slippery pulse, usually associated with vomiting, indicates an excess syndrome in most cases, whereas small, weak and uneven pulse often associated with acid regurgitation, indicates a deficiency syndrome. Floating and moderate pulse suggests a curable case, large but weak pulse suggests the deficiency of qi, and deep, uneven and small pulse indicates deficiency of blood.

Foamy vomitus is the symbol of depletion of the body fluid, especially exhaustion of the stomach yin. Vomiting with egg-white-like water or cold clear and diluted water is mostly contributable to weakness of the spleen yang.

III THERAPEUTIC PRINCIPLE

TCM treatment should be conducted based on the principle of treating different cases according to different symptoms and signs by adopting traditional anticancer drugs with modification. Supporting the kidney and spleen is the most fundamental therapeutic principle.

As the spleen dominates transformation and transportation and its large collateral distributes over the chest, sinking of the spleen qi and upward adverse flow of the stomach qi are ascribed for dysphagia, while, as the kidney rules the body fluid and its steaming function controls both the defecation and urination, the liver and kidney are responsible for the closing of the lower orifice due to failure of body fluid to nourish it. Thos for cases with dysfunction of the spleen and stomach, treatment should be directed at warming up the middle-jiao and removing dampness from the spleen to promote the ascending and descending movement of qi; while for cases with disturbance of the liver and the kidney, treatment should aim at promoting production of body fluid and removing dryness, relieving the depression of the liver qi and dispelling pathogenic wind. Deficiency of the stomach yin and the ensuing production of dryness due to sparcity of the kidney water should be treated, first of all, with drugs enriching water and nourishing the kidney. And exuberance of dampness and deficiency of the spleen caused by insufficiency of the kidney yang should be treated with drugs supporting the heart yang simultaneously. In a work, the therapeutic principle is to purge the excessive pathogen, nourish the deficient vital qi and moist dryness. Prescriptions with drastic purgative action, high toxic pungent or aromatic in taste and warm or dry in nature should be avoided.

(1) Treating the primary cause: The final purpose of treating carcinoma lies in controlling the further development of the tumor mass, and destroying and removing the tumor lesion. Though several years of selection, the authors have found handreds of Chinese herbs with the action of anticancer, which later were made into simple or patent drugs.

(2) Emergent relief of blockage of the esophagus: When the esophagus is sudden blocked and even water can not enter, first aid must be given to relieve the emergent condition. Blockage of the esophagus can be induced very easily by

emotional disturbance or the sudden aggravation of the condition, even under normal conditions. But it can also be relieved within several hours or 1-2 days by oral administration of Double Redness Liquid in combination with acupuncture and fluid transfusion.

(3) Supporting the vital qi: The treatment meassures mentioned in the ancient medical books are mostly based on the understanding that the disease is due to excessive qi, blood, phlegm or fire. According to clinical observation, however, the understanding is wrong, as most of the cases are the aged and weak in constitution and the disease is consumptive. For cases due to pathogenic accumulation in the three yang channels, the treatment should be to support the spleen and stomach first, then to enrich blood, remove dryness and clear away heat from the upper and middle-jiao. On the other hand, because the maligancy may be related to the enviromental pollution, improper diet, or the gradual infiltration of an ulcer or fistuls, the disease is also considered a surgical condition in TCM. Correspondingly, the treatment should be directed at clearing away heat, removing toxic materials and removing dampness. Drugs applicable include: Jin Yin Huan (Flos Lonicerae), Lian Qiao (Fructus Forsythiae), Dang Gui (Rhizoma Angelicae Sinensis), Bai shao (Radix Paeniae Abla), Sheng Di (Radix Rehmannia), Mai Dong (Radix Asparagi), Shi Hu (Herba Dendrobii), Ou Zhi (Lotus Juice), Li Zhi (Pear Juice), Luo Bo Zhi (Turnip Juice), Gan Zhi (Surgarcane Juice), Lu Zhi (Juice of reed rhizome), Zhu Ru (Caulis Bambusae in Taeniam), Pi Pa Ye (Folium Eri obotryae), Shi Chang Pu (Rhizome Acori Graminei), Zhu Li (Bamboo Juice), Jiu Zhi (Juice of Allii Taberosi), Mu Li (Concha Ostreae), Ge Fen (Powder of Gecko) and Qing dai (Indigo Naturalis). Patients should drink more milk. For cases with unsmooth flow of qi through the esophagus.

Qing Yang Qi Ge Decoction (Decoction for Relieving Stricture of Esophagus) or Qi Ge Decoction (Decoction for Esophagus Cancer) Should be adopted; for cases with consumption of yin due to heat from longstanding stagnation marked by severe dryness symtoms. Zi Yin Jiu Fen Decoction (Decoction for Nourishing Yin to Reduce Fire) should be selected; and for cases with stagnation of qi and hyperactivity of the liver marked by chest distension and upward adverse flow of qi, general weakness and exuberance of dampness, Shen Zhe Pei Qi Decoction (Ginseng and Ochra Haematium Decoction for Invigorating Qi) is to be adopted.

IV DIFFERENTIATION AND
TREATMENT OF COMMON SYNDROME

Although there is no uniform typing of esophageal carcinoma, the available typing is much the same with only minor differences. They mainly reflect the different aspects of various syndromes which occur in cetrain stages of cancer development , to facilitate therapy by syndrome differentiation. 5 types are summed up as follows.

1. Stagnancy of qi and liver type: Corresponding to stage 0-1.

Main symptoms and signs: there is no apparent difficulty in swallowing. Occasionally patient feels burning pain in esophagus during food ingestion, or retrosternal depressed sensation accompanied with epigastric flatulence, belching, tongue normal or slightly dark, with thin white coating, X-ray and other examination all show signs of early stage.

Therapeutic principle: Dissolving the stagnation of liver and qi.

Recipe:

Poria	15g
Rhizoma Atractylodis Macrocephalae	12g
Radix Paeoniae Alba	10g
Radix Angelicae Sinensis	9g
Radix Bupleuri	9g
Radix Glycyrrhizae	4g
Pericarpium Citri Reticulatae	9g
Caulis Perillae	10g
Cortex Magnoliae Officinalis	12g
Radix Codonopsis	15g
Radix Sophorae Tonkinensis	12g
Herba Oldenlandiae Diffusae	24g

Add or subtract drugs according to existing symptoms.

2. Simple dysphagia type: Corresponds to stage I-II or early cases of stage III.

Main symptoms and signs: No apparent symptoms except the feeling of obstruction when eating. The majority belong to medullary or fungoid type or are unilaterally involved, tongue slightly dark, thin white or thin yellow coating, thready pulse.

Therapeutic principle: Regulating the qi and relaxing the middle warmer, relieving obstruction and dispersing lumps.

Recipe:

Rhizoma Dioscorreae Bulbiferae	15g
Semen Impatientis	15g
Radix Curcumae	12g
Fructus Aurantii	9g
Spica Prunellae	15g
Herba Rabdosiae	15g
Poria	15g
Cortex Magnoliae Officinalis	10g
Fructus Citri Sarcodactylis	10g
Radix Aucklandiae	9g
Radix Codonopsis	12g
Rhizoma Dioscoreae	12g

Xinghuang Tablet: 3 to 4 tablets, three times per day.

3. Blood stasis with pain type: Corresponding to medullary type of advanced stage with majority of ulcerative type.

Main symptoms and signs: Dysphagia accompanied with fixed chest and back pain, especially aggravated during swallowing, ozostomia, dry, bitter, hot sensation in mouth, some constipation, resulting from the invasion of the tumor into the esophageal adventitia and its surroundings or the occurrence of cancerous ulceration and inflammation. Tongue dark with yellow greasy or thick yellow coating, slippery or deep and uneven pulse.

Therapeutic principle: Dissolving stasis and alleviating pain, clearing evil heat and detoxicating.

Recipe:

Flos Lonicerae	10g
Radix Scutellariae	9g
Rhizoma Coptidis	9g
Fructus Trichosanthis	18g
Radix Ophiopogonis	10g

Rhizoma Anemarrhenae	12g
Radix Sophorae Tonkinensis	15g
Radix Pseudostellariae	12g
Poria	15g
Radix Paeoniae Rubra	10g
Olibanum	6g
Myrrha	15g
Radix Astragali	15g
Radix Clematidis	10g
Radix Notoginseng	1.5g

Xinhuang Tablet: 3 to 4 tablets per day, to be taken after meals.

Zhentong Jiedu Liquid: 0.1% procaine 100ml, streptomycin 2mg or gentamycin sulfate 240,000 units, dexamethasone 1.5mg, ephedrine 60mg and belladonna tincture 3ml mixed, 10ml 3 or 4 times per day.

4. Asthenia spleen with phlegm and dampness type: The majority of this type belong to medullary or constrictive type of esophageal carcinoma, or cardiac carcinoma, all in the advanced stage.

Main symptoms and signs: Dysphagia, excessive sputum(expectorating filiform mucus), no sense of taste, preference for warmth and dryness, aversion to cold, emaciation, pale complexion, edema of lower limbs occurs in severe cases, tongue pale or dark cynotic, with indentations from teeth on edge, white greasy and wet coating, weak pulse.

Therapeutic principle: Warming and invigorating the spleen, dissolving the stagnation and expelling the dampness.

Recipe:

Radix Codonopsis	12g
Radix Astragali	15g
Radix Aucklandiae	9g
Pericarpium Citri Reticulatae	9g
Rhizoma Pinelliae Ternata	9g
Rhizoma Zingiberis	9g
Fructus Jujube	6g
Scolopendra	3g
Rhizoma Atractylodis Macrocephalae	12g

Radix Notoginseng	1. 5g
Flos Inulae	9g
Haematitum	12g
Flos Caryophylli	6g
Fructus Evodiae	9g

Add or subtract drugs according to the existing symptoms.

5. Exhaustion of yin-yang type: Corresponding to late stage III or stage IV.

Main symptoms and signs: Dysphagia unable to drink, malnutrition, qi and blood extremely exhausted, severe dehydration, emaciation, dry mouth and throat, oliguria, and constipation. Tongue dark crimson and dry, with or without coating, body of tongue withered, in serious case curled up, faint and fast pulse.

Therapeutic principle: Nourishing yin and yang, relieving obstruction and dispersing lumps.

Recipe:

Radix Ophiopogonis	12g
Radix Glehniae	10g
Herba Dendrobii	12g
Rhizoma Gynostemmatis Pentaphylli	12g
Rhizoma Polygonati Odorate	10g
Poria	15g
Succus Bambusae	10-20ml
Radix Astragali	15g
Radix Rehmanniae	12g
Fructus Cannabis	9-12g
Herba Cistanches	12g
Rhizoma Polygonati	12g
Herba Scutellariae Barbarae	24g
Herba Oldenlandiae Diffusae	30g
Herba Solanii Lyrati	24g
Radix Panacis Quinquefolii	6g

(or Radix Panacis Quiquefolii Lateralis 6g)

Kaiguan powder:

Calculus Bovis	1.5g
Moschus	1.5g
Lignum Aquilariae Resinatum	9g
Lapis Micae Aureus	9g
Sal Ammoniaci	9g
Sal Nitri	30g
Borax	50g
Borneolum Syntheticum	9g

All to be ground into powder, keep in sealed bottle, 1.5g of Kaiguan Powder is dissolved in the mouth, 5 to 10 times per day.

6. Excess of fire type:

Main symptoms and sign: Weakness of the general condition, severe pain in the chest and back, irritability. Dark red tongue with smooth, or crimson dry tongue, with yellow coating. Taut thready or thready rapid pulse, or taut rapid and strenous.

Therapeutic principle: Nourishing yin to reduce fire, normalizing the function of the liver by regulating the flow of qi.

Recipe:

(1) Si Jun Zi Tang (Decoction with Four Noble Drugs), add Radix Scutellariae, Rhizoma Coptidis.

(2) Qi Qi Tang (Decoction for Combined Pathogens)

Radix Ginseng

Radix Glycyrrhizae

Rhizoma Pinelliae

Cortex Cinnamomi

Rhizoma Zingiberis Recens

V TCM THERAPY COORDINATING
WITH MODERN MEDICINALTREATMENT

1. Preoperative treatment: Correct the imbalance of yin and yang by syndrome differentiation, when the predominance is not clear. Treatment for strengthening the body resistence is proposed to reduce the side effects of the

surgery and to promote rehabilitation. The prescription generally used is:

Radix Codonopsis	15g
Rhizoma Atractylodis Macrocephalae	12g
Poria	12g
Radix Glycyrrhizae	3g
Radix Pseudostellariae	15g
Radix Glehniae	10g
Rhizoma Polygonati	12g
Fructus Ligustici Lucidi	12g
Radix Astragali	15g
Herba Oldenlandiae Diffusae	24g
Flos Lonicerae	10g
Herba Solanii Lyrati	24g

In addition, Radix Ginseng or Radix Panacis Quinquefolii 6g after boiling, is given alone or is combined with other Chinese herbal medicines for 2 to 3 consecutive days prior to surgery.

2. Postoperative treatment: Owing to the traumatic injury, complications resulting from surgery, and a certain degree of danger, implementing postoperative TCM management based on syndrome differentiation can markedly reduce postoperative complications and sequelae. Therapy should begin 3 to 4 days after surgery. the basic prescription is:

Radix Glehniae	10g
Radix Ophiopogonis	10g
Poria	12g
Rhizoma Polygonati	12g
Radix Astragali	15g
Radix Pseudostellariae	15g
Radix Codonopsis	12g
Fructus Trichosanthis	24g
Fructus Hordei Germinatus	24g
Endothelium Corneum Gigeriae Galli	9g
Radix Ginseng or Radix Panacis Quinquefolii	4-6g

Add or substract drugs according to syndrome differentiation.

3. Combining radiotherapy and TCM

The chief factors causing failure of radiotherapy for esophageal carcinoma are: local relapse and inability to control the focus, side effects due to radiotherapy, such as, radiation myelopathy, bronchitis, pneumonia, esophagitis, ulceration, perforation or inhibition of bone marrow, and impairment of the immunological functions. TCM therapy based on syndrome differentiation can enhance the immunological functions, reduce side effects, improve the microcirculation, increase the number of anaerobic cells, and escalate sensitivity to radiotherapy. The prescription generally used is:

Flos Lonicerae	9g
Rhizoma Coptidis	6g
Rhizoma Gynostemmatis Pentaphylli	15g
Poria	12g
Radix Rehmanniae	10g
Radix Astragali	15g
Rhizoma Atractylodis Macrocephalae	12g
Radix Pseudostellariae	15g
Radix Salviae Miltiorrhizae	12g
Pericarpium Citri Reticulatae	9g
Polyporus	15g
Radix Glycyrrhizae	5g
Herba Oldenlandiae Diffusae	24g
Rhizoma Dioscoreae	12g
Fructus Amomi Rotundus	9g
Fructus Ligustici Lucidi	12g

Add or substract drugs according to symptoms presented.

Combined treatment of TCM and WM should be applied according to the existing side effects, administration of antibiotics, maintaining the water and electrolyte balance, supplementing proteins, vitamins and glucose, and use of drugs for improving microcirculation, all of which are equaly important. When severe side reactions appear, radiotherapy should be suspended until reactions subside.

4. Prevention and treatment of reactions to chemotherapy

Due to the difference in chemical toxicity and individual differences in sensitivity and tolerance, reactions may vary a great deal. Some may reveal no reaction to the chemical, while others may have serious reactions although they have received only one or two regular doses. There is no strict rule for completing the whole therapeutic dosage, the chemicals selected, and method for administering dosage, or periods of interruption, as the total course will vary with each individual and with different ailments. Reactions can not be advoided, and should never be left untreated, or the patient's condition will deteriorate.

Representative prescription for reactions: Since the common reaction is injury of normal cells by toxicity, with an ensuing imbalance of body functions, the treatment should be the increass of health energy, detoxication, and repair of injuries to rectify the deviation. For this purpose, There is a prescription Yiqi Buxue Jianpi Decoction, indicated for every type of reaction. The ingredients are:

Radix Astragali	15-30g
Radix Codonopsis	15-18g
Radix Atractylodis Macrocephalae	12g
Poria	12g
Radix Glycyrrhizae	4.5g
Radix rehmanniae Prepatata	10g
Fructus Lycii	12g
Radix Polygoni Multiflon	12g
Rhizoma Polygonati	10g
Fructus Ligustri Lucidi	15g
Radix Glehniae	10g
Radix Ophiopogonis	10g
Caulis Spatholobi	24g
Semen Euryales	12g
Rhizoma Dioscorea	12g

Decoct the above ingredients with water three times. To be adminstered along with chemotherapy and at interals between therapeutic courses, until symptoms disappeat. As the prescription indicateds, it regulates gastrointestinal functions, promotes hemopoetic function , protects the heart, liver, kidney endocrines and cells from being injured and at the same time improves immunity.

This prescription can generally be taken for a longer period, without altering the ingredients. However, modifications need to be made, should manifestations change, depending on the syndromes, disease and according to the affected organ.

Modifications according to symptoms:

Nausea and vomiting: Add Fructus Evodia, Rhizoma Coptidis, Rhizoma Pinelliae prepared with ginger, Caulis Bambusae in Taeniam, Calyx Kaki, Flos Caryophylli; decrease sufficiently Caulis sqatholobi, Radix Polygoni Multiflori.

Abdominal distension: Add Radix Aucklandiae Pericarpium Citri Reticulatae, Fructus Citri Sarcodactylis, Massa Medicata Fermentata; decrease sufficiently, Radix Ophiopogonis, Caulis Spatholobi.

Abdominal pain: Add Rhizoma Corydalis, Herba Chelidonii, Radix Linderae.

Loss of appetite: Add Endothelium Corneum Gigeriae Galli, Fructus Hordei Geriminatus, Fructus Setariae Germinatus, Fructus Crataegi, Massa Medicata Fermentata, Semen Euryales, Semen Nelumbinis; decrease sufficiently Radix Rehmanniae Prepatata, Fructus Psoraleae, Caulis Spatholobi, Radix Polygoni Multiflori.

Dry tongue and mouth: Add Herba Dendrobii, Rhizoma Anemarrheneae, Rhizoma Polygonati Odorati, Nodus Nelumbinis Rhizomatis, Radix Scrophulariae, Rhizoma Imperatae, Radix Rehmanniae, Radix Asparagi, Radix Pseudostellariae, Succus Bambusae, decrease sufficiently Radix Astragali, Radix Codonopsis, Radix Rhehmanniae Preparata, Radix Polygonati Multiflori, Semen Euryales, Rhizoma Dioscoreae.

Constipation: Add Fructus Cannabis, Fructus Trichosanthis Radix Rhei, Herba Cistanches. Folium Sennae; decrease sufficiently Fructus Psolarae, Radix Polygonati Multiflori, Radix Rehmanniae Preparata, Radix Codonopsis, Semen Euryales, Rhizoma Dioscoreae.

Diarrhea: Add Pericarpium Papaveris, Herba Chelidonii, Rhizoma Coptidis, Cortex Fraxini, Cortex Magnoliae Officinalis; decrease sufficiently Radix Ophiopogonis, Radix Glehniae, Caulis Spatholobi.

Flat taste in Mouth with Cold Saliva(cold spleen and stomach): Add Rhizoma Zingiberis, Fructus Amomi Rotundus, Flos Caryophylli, Fructus Jujubae, Cortex Cinnamomi, Radix Aconiti Lateralis Preparata, Radix ginseng; decrease sufficiently Radix Ophiopogonis, Radix Glehniae, Rhizoma Polygonati, Fructus Ligustri Lucidi, Caulis Spatholobi.

Insomnia: Add Semen Ziziphi Spinosae, Fructus schisandrae, Semen Platy-cladi, Concha Ostreae, Caulis Polygoni Multiflori; decrease sufficiently Rhizoma Polygonati, Radix Astragal.

Anasarca: Add Semen Plantaginis, Rhizoma Alismatis, Poria, Caulis Clematidis Armandii, Placenta Hominis, Semen Pharbitidis; decrease sufficiently Radix Ophiopogonis, Radix Glehniae, Fructus Ligustri Lucidi.

Anamia: Add Radix Angelicae Sinensis, Placenta Hominis, Radix Astra-gali, with Caulis Spatholobi in heavy doses.

Fever: Add Herba Atremisia Scoporiae, Flos Lonicerae, Niuhuang Jiere Powder, Xinhuang Tablet, Pianzihuang; decrease sufficiently Radix Rehmanni-ae Preparata, Caulis Spatholobi, radix Polygoni Multiflori.

Coughing: Add Bulbus Fritillariae Cirrhosae, Flos Farfarae, Radix Asteris Semen Armeniacae Amarum, Folium Enobotryae, Herba Houttuyniae; decease sufficiently Radix Rehemanniae Preparata, Radix Polygonati Multiflori, Caulis Spatholobi, Rhizoma Polygonati.

Hematochezia: Add Cacumen Platycladi Radix Sanguisorbae, Radix Noto-ginseng, Crinis Carbonisatus, Nodus Nelumbinis, Rhizomatis Carbouisatus, Herba Callicarpae pseudoculatae, Colla Corii Asini; decrease sufficiently Radix Rehmanniae Preparata, radix Polygoni Multiflori.

Skin Lesion (rash, erythema, exfoliative dermatitis, alopecia): Add Radix Rehmanniae, Cortex Moutan, Fructus Cornii, Herba Cistanches. For exfoliative dermatitis, use 100 ml of tea seed oil, 100mg of desamethaxone poeder, for local application.

Pulmonary Fibrosis: Add Radix Ginseng, Radix Salviae Miltiorrhizae, Rhi-zoma Chuangxiong, Flos Lonicerae, Xinhuang Tablet, along with antibiotic, prednisone, polysacharides from Poria and Polyporus, decrease sufficiently Caulis Spatholobi, Rhizoma Polygonati, radix Rehmanniae Prepatata.

Inhibition of Bone Marrow: Add Radix Ginseng Placenta Homins Cornce Cervi Pantotichum, Herba Epimedii, Radix Angelicae Sinensis, Fructus Corni Gelatinum, Collacorii Asini, colla Cornus Cervi, with a heavy dose of Radix As-tragali polysacharides from Polyporus and Poria Injection.

Nervoun system affected: Add semen Juglandis, Fructus Corni Lac Regis Apis, add heavy dose of Eructus Lycii, Radix Ginseng, Radix Rehmanniae, Se-men Cuscutae Radix Morindae Officinalis, Radix Salviae Miltiorrhizae along with

ATP, B 12, B, B6, co-enzyme Q10, Cytochrome C, dexamethasone; decrease sufficiently Caulis Spatholobi, Radix rehmanniae Preparata, Rhizoma Atractylodis Macrocephalae, Rhizoma dioscoreae.

Anemia: Add Radix Angelicae Sinenisis, Rhizoma Chuanxiong, Radix Salviae Miltiorrhizae, Fructus Corni, Herba Leonuri.

Oligosperima: Add Herba Epimedii, Semen Cuscutae, Semen Trigonellae, Herba Cistanches, Lac Regis Apis, Radix Ginseng, Cornu Cervi Pantotrichum; decrease sufficiently Caulis Spatholobi, Radix Polygoni Multiflori, Rhizoma Polygonati, Rhizoma Dioscoreae.

Fu Zheng Pei Ben Principle (FZPB) therapy for side effects from chemotherapy is not applied exclusively by TCM. Supportive measures of western medicine also have a form of FZPB. When serious side effects occur, western methods when fully exploited, yield definite and timely results. Generally, when there are only mild side effects or no side effects, TCM can be applied. If the side effects are serious, integrated methods should be used, including blood transfusion for bone marrow inhibition, antibiotics or hormones for infection. Bone marrow or thrombocytes transfusion, with light doses of ACTH can be administered, when condition permit.

When nutrition is insufficient, protein hydrolysate, glucose, and amino acids should be administered. When edema occurs, due to low immunity or low plasmal protein, human albumin and dried plasma should be given. If the patient vomits, manifesting dehydration and water electrolyte disturbance, an ample supply of fluid, electrolytes, vitamen B_6 and C should be prescribed and anti-nausea remedies, such as paspertin, should be given. Analgesics for pain, hypnotics for insomnia, and other helpful measures should also be considered.

5. Strengthening the effect of chemotherapy

Clinicallly, FZ drugs, including extracted polyssacharides, when given with chemicals, not only alleviate side effects, they also strengthen the therapeutic effect of the chemicals. A hospital reported 44 cases of carcinoma of the lung were treated with polyssacharides from Polyporus Umbellitus, and another 19 cases treated simply with chemicals as control. Results showed, in the experimental group, the rate of tumor shrinkage and two yeat survival rate, were all higher than the control group. This combination stimulated the appetite, increased body weight and upgraded cellular immunity. When carboxyl-methyl-poria polysacharides was included along with MFV chemotherapy, then compared with simple MFV therapy, in all 20 cases of advanced carcinoma of the stomach, I found all above indices for effectiveness seemed better in the first group. In the experimental group the sufvival rate was eight months longer. 81 cases of late stage carcinoma of the stmach were treated at Beijing TCM Hospital using shengxue decoction as adjuvant to chemotherapy. Results revealed in the experimental group, showed the incidence of general and digestive reactions as apparently lower while body weight increased, serum gastrin contents werte higher, when compared with the simple chemotherapy group, protection of bone marrow and function of the macrophage also improved.

Chapter Fifteen
Carcinoma of Stomach

Carcinoma of stomach frequently seen in clinic is one tumor of the digestive tract and has a high incidence. Statistics from 38 hospitals repored an average morbidity of 48. 4% and 46. 7% respectiively being the second highest incidence of carcinomas of the digestive tract. Men are more frequently affected than women and the morbidity of the former (74%) is 3 times that of the latter (26%). The predilection sites of the disease involve mainly the pyloric antrum and the lesser curvature of stomach (25-75%), rarely the fundus (15%) and cardia (10%). At its initial stage, no conspicuous symptoms and signs can be detected and thus it is prone to be misdiagnosed as peptic ulcer or gastritis. Usually it has progressed to the advanced stage when its typical manifestations appear and the diagnosis is ascertained. And as a result of the delayed diagnosis and the earlier occurrence of metastasis, the possibility of excision and the 3-5 years postoperative survival rate are comparatively low. For this reason, carcinoma of stomach should be listed among the corcinomas to be first conquered.

Carcinoma of stomach, as a particular disease, is not recorded in the ancient Chinese medical literature. However, the terms used to describe a kind of disease . similar to carcinoma of stomach such as Fan Wei (regurgitation of food). Wei Fan (adverse flow of food from the stomach), Yan (cancer), have been found. Of the five Fa (phlegmon or skin cancer)syndromes mentioned in the book Precious Works on Hygiene compiled by Mr. Dong Xuan, a lay Buddhist in the Song Dyhasty the first listed was carcinoma, which had also been discussed by many physicians throughout history. Nevertheless, those descriptions have only refered to the superficial tumors in the scope of surgical diseases in traditional Chinese medicine such as Ru Yan(breast cancer), Shen Yan (kidney cancer), Fan Hua (skin cancer), and Can Chun (carcinoma of lips). Although there was no special record on carcinomas of the internal organs miscellaneous descriptions on some internal diseases resembling carcinomas can still be found. Differentiation of types and corresponding treatment of carcinoma of stomach are just on the basis of the therapeutic principles adopted in treating Ye Ge (disphagia) and of the measures for skin disorders).

There are no obvious symptoms in the early stage, When symptoms appear, most patients are in the middle or advanced stage, which is difficult to treat. In recent years, due to the increase in technical knowledge helpful to early diagnosis, and the application of combined therapy of TCM and Western medicine, great progress in both prevention and treatment has been made.

I CLINICO-PATHOLOGICAL STAGING

Four stages of SC were designated by the National Conference on Carcinoma of the Stomach in 1977.

Stage 1 (T_{1-2} No Mo): Superficial SC without lymph node metastasis, or neoplasm in vasion of muscular layer, and lesion is less than 1/2 zonation.

Stage II ($T_3 N_0 M_0$, $T_{1-3} N_1 M_0$): superficial SC with lymph node metastasis of first station, or neoplasm has invaded the muscular layer, and lesion is less than 1 zonation; the lesion involves the serosal layer, lesion does not involve serosal layer, and the lesion exceeds 1/2 zonation; with or without lymph node metastasis to adjacent regions.

Stage III ($T_{4a} N_{0-1} M_0$): With distant metastasis of superficial lymph node or nearby metastasis of deep group lymph node, regardless of the size of neoplasm; with no lymph node metastasis, but the lesion exceeds 1 zonation, and involves the surrounding tissues.

Stage IV (M_1 and T_{4b} groups): with distant metastasis or metastasis at the hepatic portal, paraabdominal aorta, paramiddle artery of colon or radical part of mesenteric lymph node, regardless of the size of neoplasm.

II CLICICAL MANIFESTATION

1. Symptoms

The symptoms of early stage SC are not obvious. When there is a symptom, it is non-specific and often resembles chronic gastritis, gastric ptosis and duodenal bulb ulcer. When a typical symptom appears, it belongs to the advanced stage. The following symptoms are common.

Distress or pain in stomach: Frequently appears as distension or dull pain for a long period. When the neoplasm locates at the gastric antrum, influencing the duodenal function, the rhythmic hunger pain of duodenal bulb ulcer frequently occurs. Sometimes immediate relief is obtained with treatment for gastritis or peptic ulcer, so the patient is not concerned and time is lost. As the disease develops, the pain gradually increases, and becomes irregular and protracted. when the neoplasm involves the pancreas, the pain becomes sustained and radiates to the lumbar region. It is aggravated when lying flat, and relieved with the bending of the thigh, a posture inclining forward or lying prostrate.

Nausea and vomiting: Nausea occasionally occurs in early stage, but vomiting is usually caused by obstruction of the pylorus by neoplasm, it eructates gas with a foul odor, and vomitus is foul and tart putrefied food. Coffee-colored gastric content is usually vomited in the late stage. If the neoplasm is located at the lesser gastric curvature, the patient vomits without obstruction; If it is located at the gastric funfus and cardia, which causes the constricture of cardia, and dysphagia occurs.

Anorexia: It appears during the early stage of SC, causing a feeling of fullness, distension and belching after meals. this gradually becomes more aggravated. The majority of patients are disgusted by meat and fatty food and gradually become emaciated, have a pale complexion and lethargic.

Hematemesis and hematochezia: Because the surface of the neoplasm erodes, there is chronic seeping of capillary blood. The occult blood of stool is always positive. Negative conversion occasionally occurs, but remains only for a short period. Since the ulcerated carcinoma involves blood vessels, hematemesis and melena appear, and it is difficult to stop the bleeding. After the profuse bleeding stops, coffee-colored gastric content is usually vomited.

Other symptoms: Anemia is caused by acute and chronic bleeding; Partial pyloric obstruction leads to putrefied food entering the intestinal tract causing diarrhea; Protracted course of the disease impairs the Yin causing constipation; Food-intake is never enough for the neoplasm's consumption, which causes cachexia.

2. Physical signs

There are no apparent physical signs in early stage of SC, but a hard lump is palpable at the epigastrium. Gastric ptosis patient's lump is palpable around the umbilicus, is mostly mobile and in accord with breathing. If the tumor has adhered to surrounding tissues, it is immobile and large. The majority are infiltrative carcinoma, frequently located at gastric corpus and antrum. The tumor mass of cardia -fundus carcinoma is barely palpable, and when found, belongs to the advanced stage. In some SC patients of stage IV, a hard metastatic lymph node is palpable in the left supraclavicular fossa; metastatic carcinoma nodules in the pelvis are located with digital palpation. When the nodules spreads to the liver, they become enlarged, hard and have an uneven surface. As SC spreads to the peritoneum, the portal vein is compressed by the tumor mass, and causes portal hypertension or hypoproteinemia, ascites and edema of lower extremities followed electrolyte disturbance. This makes surgery difficult to perform, and will result in further complications. If TCM and Westen medicine adjustments for imbalance and disturbance are made before surgery, to create favorable conditions for surgery, postoperative complications will be reduced. some SC when in the advanced stage infiltrate adjacent organs, making them inoperable. If chemotherapy and TCM are adopted until the tumor mass shrinks, the infiltration and adhesion decreases, and palliative resection can be performed. This creates a situation permitting future combined TCM and Western therapy.

III DIFFERENTIATION AND
TREATMENT OF COMMON SYNDROME

According to the program of national coordination aggreed upon in 1985 by the professional committee of oncology, of the Chinese association for the integration of TCM and western medicine.

1. Imbalancc of liver and stomach type: Corresponding to stage I-II, in the majority of cases the focus is located at antral region of stomach, accompanied by incomplete pyloric obstruction.

Main symptoms and signs: Epigastric distention and pain, at no specific time, after meals or as hunger pain, epigastric distress, belching with fetid odor, vomiting, occasional insomnia, restlessness, conjestion of the chest, tongue red with thin yellow or white coating, faint and string-like pulse.

Therapeutic principle: Soothing the liver qi and harmonizing stomach, lowering the abnormally ascending qi and relieving the pain.

Recipe:

Radix Bupleuri	9g
Haematitum	9g
Radix Paeoniae Alba	9g
Fructus Aurantii	7g
Radix Aucklandiae	9g
Radix Codonopsis	15g
Rhizoma Atractylodis Macrocephalae	12g
Rhizoma Pinelliae	8g
Pericarpium Citri Reticulatae	9g
Poria	15g
Radix Glycyrrhizae	3g
Rhizoma Coptidis	6g
Rhizoma Cyperi	6g

Add or subtract drugs according to existing symptoms.

2. Asthenia of spleen and stomach type: Corresponding to stage II-III, with anemia, persistent positive reaction of occult blood in stool, lowering of hemoglobin.

Main symptoms and signs: Dull epigastric pain, preference for warm, aversion to cold, or disgust for fatty food, anorexia, frequent vomiting of cold fluid, cold limbs, normal or loose stool, pale complexion, sometimes edema of lower limbs is present, listlessness and exhaustion, tongue with indentations tooth around edges, white moist coating on tongue, deep and faint pulse.

Therapeutic principle: Warming the middle warmer, dispelling evil cold, invigorating the spleen and harmonizing the stomach.

Recipe : Lizhong Decoction, Liujunzi Decoction or Wuzhuyu decoction.

Rhizoma Alpiniae Officinarum	9g
Rhizoma Zingiberis	9g
Rhizoma Pinellia	9g
Radix Glycyrrhizae	3g
Rhizoma Cyperi	9g
Semen Aesculi	9g
Fructus Jujube	6g
Fructus Amomi	6g
Radix Codonopsis	15g
Poria	15g
Rhizoma Atractylodis Macrocephalae	15g

Add or subtract drugs according to existing symptoms.

3. Stagnation of qi and stasis of blood type: Corresponding to stage II-III or stage IV, with a large cancerous ulceration, or tumor has infiltrated to pancreas involving the celiacganglia, and hypercoagulability of blood.

Main symptoms and signs: Stabbing epigastric pain, with tenderness, occasional upper abdominal fullness, with palpable tumor mass, hematemesis, hematochezia or with coffee-colored vomitus, dry skin, dark purple tongue with petichia, faint or deep, faint and uneven pulse.

Therapeutic principle: Removing the stasis and promoting blood circulation, regulating the flow of qi and relieving pain.

Recipe: Taohong Siwu Decoction and Zhuyu Decoction.

Radix Angelicae Sinensis	9g
Radix Paeoniae Rubra	9g
Semen Persicae	9g
Flos Carthami	9g

Pollen Typhae	8g
Faeces Trogopterori	9g
Rhizoma Corydalis	9g
Radix Curcuumae	9g
Fructus Toosendan	9g
Cacumen Platycladi	18g
Poria	15g
Radix Ophiopogonis	10g
Radix Glehniae	10g

Add or subtract drugs according to existing symptoms.

4. Yin impaired by stomach-heat type: Corresponding to stage II-IV, characterized by the functional distubance of vegetative nerve, change in hemorheology, increase in blood viscosity.

Main symptoms and signs: Burning epigastric pain, dry mouth, anorexia, preference for cold drinks, epigastric upset, disphoria with difficulty in breathing, dry stool, red uncoated, smooth tongue with yellow or little coating, pulse slippery, faint and rapid.

Therapeutic principle: Nourishing yin, clearing up the evil heat, replenishing stomach and harmonizing middle warmer.

Recipe: Shasheng Maidong Decoction and Yangwei Decoction.

Radix Glehniae	10g
Radix Ophiopogonis	9g
Folium Bambusae	9g
Rhizoma Polygonati Odorati	9g
Herba dendrobii	9g
Rhizoma Anemarrhenae	9g
Radix Trichosanthis	9g
Radix Pseudostellariae	15g
Poria	15g
Radix Paeoniae Alba	10g
Fructus Cannabis	9g
Fructus Trichosanthi	20g

Add or subtract drugs according to existing symptoms.

5. Insufficiency of spleen with phlegm-dampness type: Occurs at various

stages of gastric carcinoma, or cardia involved with malignancy of gastic fundus, it manifests itself chiefly by inhibiting the sympathetic nerve, anemia, emaciation and malnutrition.

Main symptoms and signs: Epigastric fullness and pain, copious expectoration, loss of taste, anorexia, normal or loose stool, nausea and vomiting, dark red or light red tongue with white or yellow greasy coating, pulse slippery and faint.

Therapeutic principle: Invigorating the spleen, removing the dampness by diuresis, resolving phlegm and calming down stomach.

Recipe: Liujunzi Decoction and Erchen Decoction.

Radix Pseudostellariae	15g
Rhizoma Atractylodis Macrocephalae	15g
Poria	15g
Rhizoma Pinelliae	9g
Pericarpium Citri Reticulatae	6g
Fructus Perillae	9g
Semen Rapheni	15g
Bulbus Fritillaria Cirrhosae	9g
Semen Coicis	24g

Add or subtract drugs according to existing symptoms.

6. Both deficiency of qi and blood tyoe: Advanced stage, cachexia, hypoproteinemia, anemia

Main symptoms and signs: General weakness, palpitation, shortness of breath, vertigo and blurred vision, sallow complexion, spontaneous perspiration and night sweating, edema of limbs especially the lower limbs, pulse sunken, faint and weak, tongue pale with little coating.

Therapeutic principle: Restoring both qi and blood, strengthening body resistences and eliminating pathogenic factors.

Recipe: Bazhen Decoction and Shiquan Dabu Decoction.

Radix Codonopsis	12g
Rhizoma Atractylodis Macrocephalae	12g
Poria	15g
Radix Angelicae Sinensis	9g
Radix Paeoniae Alba	9g

Radix Rehmanniae	20g
Rhizoma Polygonati	12g
Caulis Spatholobi	18g
Radix Astragali	15g
Radix Glycyrrhizae	3g
Radix Ginseng or Radix Panacis Quinguefolium	6g

Add or subtract drugs according to existing symptoms.

Types do not stay the same during the entire course of the disease. Symptoms alter as the disease develops and medication has to be flexible. In clinical practice, it usually presents a picture of coexisting syndrome-types or intermingled deficiency and excess. It is therefore best to use clinical symptoms as a basis for syndrome differentiation and typing. Efficacy is enhanced when the patient is treated according to syndrome differentiation at the time, adding medicinal plants with anti-cancer function.

Shi et al divided this affection into three types: The yin or yang nature or the disease must be first distinguished. If it is a syndrome caused by insufficiency of yang and marked by pale complexion, aversion to cold, pale tongue proper and loose stool, the principle for the treatment should be to strengthen the spleen to reinforce yang and to aid Mingmen in its steaming function, by the aid of promoting discharge of the tubid with drugs pungent in taste and hot in nature; if it is a syndrome due to yin deficiency and blood dryness, the method of nourishing yin to suppress yang supported by relieving fullness sensation with drugs pungent in taste and slippery in nature and by replenishing vital qi with drugs sweet in taste and moist in nature should be employed, being sure not to use drugs pungent in taste and dry in nature lest the body fluids be consumed or those intense hot in nature lest the yin be depleted; if it is a syndrome caused by deficiency of both qi and blood, the method of tonifying qi and blood should be adopted; in the case of vomiting due to obstruction of the lumps, drugs with the action of removing blood stasis and promoting the downward flow of the stomach qi should be administered to prevent the gastrointestinal tract from being obstructed. What is more critical is that the prolonged illness will cause sparcity of the vital qi, so, during the whole course of treatment, vital qi must be prevented from being further consumed and should be further strengthened to remove toxic materials.

(1) Depression of qi of the liver and spleen, blood stasis and dryness:

Main symptoms and signs: This type is marked by flushed face or dim complexion, dark and purplish tongue with yellowish thick gready coating, or crimson and melena.

Therapeutic principle: Activiting the circulation of qi and blood in the Jueyin and Yangming channels to lessen the depression of the liver qi, aided by supporting the vital qi, and reinforcing the stomach yin.

Recipe:

Radix Angelicae Sinensis	12g
Radix Paeoniae Alba	12g
Rhizoma Cyperi	10g
Exocarpium citri Reticulatea	10g
Rhizoma Pinelliae	10g
Poria	10g
Caulis Bambusae in Taeniam	10g
Folium Eriobotryae	10g
Herba Dendrobii	10g
Radix Curcumae	10g

In the case of constipation, Da Huang (Rhizoma Rhei) 6 g (This drug should be added to the decoction when the other ingrtedients have been decocted some time and is used to break down the accumulation of pathogenic factors, once the effects of the drug appear, its administration should be stopped. Be sure not to apply the drug for a prolonged time) should be added; for case with unimpaired constitution, Liang Tou Jian (Rhizoma Anemones Raddeanae) 30 g (This drug has the effect of disintegrating lumps in the abdominal cavity), San Leng (Rhizoma Sparganii) 9g, E Zhu (Rhizoma Zedoariae) 9g, Yan Hu (rhizoma Corydalis) 10g, Dan Shen (Radix Salviae Miltiorrhizae) 10g can be selected to modify the prescription. Treatment of the disease in the advanced stage should be dominated by drugs to enhance vital qi, or reinforce the spleen and stomach, supported by the drugs made from insects or worms, the prescription to be administered is Ba Zhen Tang (Decoction of Eight Precious Ingredients) plus Wu Gong (Scolopendra) 9g, Di Bie Chong (Eupolyphaga seu Steleophaga) 9g , Di Long (Lumbricus) 9g, Sheng Shui Zhi (Hirudo) 9g, and Meng Chong (Tabanus) 9g, which can be administered alternately, by the way of 3 to 5 doses of tonics followed by 1 dose of purgatives, in accordance with the changes of pathogensis.

(2) Retention of cold dampness due to hypofunction of the spleen-yang:

Main symptoms and signs: Sallow and withered complexion, lassitude, indigestion, salivation without sour, bitter or fetid smell, or even vomiting containing the food taken the previous morning, loss of appetite, loose stool, pale tongue, and taut tense pulse.

Therapeutic principle: Strengthen the spleen-yag, supplemented by removing the turbid and the obstruction in the stomach with drugs pungent in taste and hot in nature.

Recipe: Li Zhong Tang (Decoction for Regulating the Function of the Middle-jiao), Wu Zhu Yu Tang (Fructus Evodiae Decoction), Bu Zhong Yi Qi Tang (Decoction for Reinforcing the Middle-jiao and Replenishing Qi) and Wei Ling Tang (Stomach Decoction with Poria). In the case with dampness in the lower-jiao and dryness in the upper-jiao. Lian Li Tang (Decoction for Reinforcing the Function of the Middle-jiao with Coptis) can be adopted, depending on patients'conditions. In the case of more dampness, Zhu Ling (Polyporus Umbellatus), Ze xie (Rhizoma Alismatis) 9g can be added, and in the case of more cold, Fu Zi (Radix Aconiti Praeparata) 3g, Gui Xin (Cortex Cinnamomi) 6g can be added. Furthermore, the drugs to be selected also include Sha RN (Fructus Amomi) 6g, Sheng Ban Xia (Rhizoma Pinelliae) 9g, Ding Xiang (Flos Caryophylli) 9g and Yi Zhi RN (Fructus Alpiniae Oxyphyllae) 10g. When yang qi begins to revive, drugs for nourishing yin and enriching blood, such as RN Shen (Radix Ginseng) 1. 5g, Shen Yao (Rhizoma Dioscoreae) 18g, Lian Zi (Semen Nelumbinis) 10g, Wu Mei (Fructus Mume) 6g, Da Zao (Fructus Ziziphi Jujubae) 4g, Nuo Mi (Semen Oryzae Glutinosae) 15g, Gan Cao (Radix Glycyrrhizae) 3g, Dang Gui (Radix Angelicae sinensis) 10g, and Shao Yao (Radix Paeoniae) 10g should be added.

At the advanced stage, deficiency of both yin and yang often appears as a result of the excessive salivation due to yang insufficiency and the subsequent loss of the body fluids. Thus, the therapeutic principle, replenishing both yin and yang to coordinate the balance betwen them, should be employed, and Ba Wei Di Huang Tang (Decoction for Invigorationg the Kidney Qi), Ba Zhen Tang (Decoction with Eight Precious Ingredients) are the decoctions to be selected. If the vital qi is about to be depleted, Ginseng Powder should be taken with water. In the case of vomiting, constipation, inability to take food caused by obstruction of the upper part of the stomach, supporting measures such as fluid transfusion can be taken. If necessary, surgical fistulation or reconstruction of the stomach can be conducted.

(3) Consumption of stomach yin:

Main symptoms and signs: Wan and sallow face, dry throat, dry and tarry stool, incessant dull pain with a cutting feeling in the stomach, crimson tongue without coating, rapid swift or rapid thready forceless pulse.

Therapeutic principle: Nourish yin with drugs sour in taste, supported by relieving fullness sensation with drugs pungent in taste and slippery in nature.

Recipe:

Radix Adenophorae Strictae	30g
Radix Salviae Miltiorrhizae	15g
Radix Ophiopogonis	9g
Fructus Mume	9g
Folium Eriobotryae	9g
Herba Dendrobii	10g
Caulis Bambusae in Taeniam	10g
Pericarpium Trichosanthis	10g
Pericarpium Citri Reticulatae	10g
Radix glycyrrhizae	3g

The alternative drugs are: Bamboo juice 20ml , Zhi Mu (Rhizoma Anemarrhenae)9g, Xing ren (Semen Armeniacae Amarum) 9g, Suan Zao RN (Semen Ziziphi Spinosae) 15g, Mu Gua (Frustus Chaenomelis) 15g, Shi Shuang (Pruina Kaki) 60g.

For cases with upward adverse flow of qi, Ban Xia (Rhizoma Pinelliae) should be used as a adjuvant drug. For cases with chest distension and poor appetite powder of Bai Jiang Xing(Lignum Santali Alba) or powder of Chen Xiang (Lingum Aquilariae) should be administered to be taken with water.

(4) Heteropathy:

(1) Fullness sensation and dull pain in the upper abdomen: Administer combined Bu Zhong Yi Qi Tang, (Decoction for Reinforcing the Middle-jiao and Invigoration Qi) and Ping Wei San (Powder for Regulating the Function of Stomach) with modifications for the deficiency type; combined Ge Xia Zhu Yu

Tang (Decoction for Dissipating Blood Stasis Under Diaphragm) and Ping Wei San (Powder for Regulating the Function of Stomach) for the excess-type; combined Li Zhong Tang (Decoction for Regulating the Function of Middle-jiao) and Wu Zhu Yu Tang (Fructus Evodiae Decoction) for the cold-type; and Yang Wei Tang (Decoction for Nourishing the Stomach) plus drugs with the action of removing blood stasis, activating the flow of blood and clearing away pathogenic heat for the heat-type.

(2) Vomiting:

Vomiting of cold type can be treated with Wu Zhu Yu Tang (Fructus Evodiae Decoction), Da Chai Hu Tang (Major Pinellina Tuber Decoction, especially effective for vomiting with vomitus containing the food eaten the previous morning).

Vomiting of heat type can be treated with Ju Pi Zhu Ru Tang (Tangerine Peel and Bamboo Shavings Decoction), combination of Chai Ping Tang (Minor Bulpleurum Decoction with Powder Pepetic), Yang Wei Tang (Decoction for Nourishing the Stomach) or by taking the decoction of Mao Gen (Rhizoma Imperatae) or the decoction of Lu Gen (Rhizoma Phargmitis) in small amout at short intervals to clear away heat from the spleen and nourish the stomach yin.

Vomiting of deficiency type can be treated with decoction of Sha RN (Fructus Amomi), Ban Xia Tang (Pinellia Tuber Decoction), Li Zhong Tang (Decoction for Regulation the Function of Replenishing Qi) and Shen Zhe Pei Qi Tang (Decoction with radix Ginseng and Ochra Haematitum for Replenishing Qi) to warm up the middle-jiao, strengthen the spleen and promote digestion.

Vomition of excess type can be treated with Jin Gui Fu Ling Ze Xie Tang(Decoction containing Poria and Rhizoma Alismatis) with Bai Zhu (Rhizoma Atractylodis Macrocephalae)removed and Ban Xia (Rhizoma Pinelliae)and Sheng Jiang (Rhizoma Zingiberis Reçens) added to remove accumulated dampness pathogens.

(3) Hematochezia: Administer Huang Tu Tang (Decoction of Baked Yellow Earth) plus Notoginseng powder, Xian He Cao (Herba Agrimoniae), Qian Cao (Radix Rubiae), Xue Yu Tang (Crinis Carbonisatus) or Pao Jiang Tang (Baked Ginger Carbonisatus) according to patients' conditions, or Bu Zhong Yi Qi Tang (Decoction for Reinforcing Middle-jiao and Replenishing Qi) together with drugs to stop bleeding for deficiency-cold type; and Gen Gen Qin Lian Tang

(Decoction of Puerariae, Scutellaria and Coptis) plus Notoginseng powder and Qian Cao (Radix Rubiae) for excess heat-type.

(5) Selection of prescriptions:

For the cases with fullness and distension due to stagnation of qi in the stomach. Ping Wei San (Pepetic Power) plus Huo Xiang (Herba Agastachis) and Sha RN (Fructus Amomi) should be selected.

For the case with weakness of qi of middle-jiao, Si Jun Zi Tang (Decoction of Four Noble Drugs) plus Huang Qi(Radix Astragali seu Hedysari), Ju Hong (Exocarpium Citri Reticulatae) and Sha RN (Fructus Amomi) should be selected.

For the cases with continuous salivation after food intake follow by vomiting. Si Jun Zi Tang (Decoction of Four Noble Drugs) plus Ding Xiang (Flos Caryophylli), Huo Xiang (Herba Agastachis), or Huo Xiang An Wei San (Agastachis Power for Calming Stomach) should be selected.

For the cases with fullness and distension feeling over the chest and feeling of obstruction in the throat. Wu Xing (Radix Aucklandiae), Sha RN (Fructus Amomi), Zhi Shi (Fructus Aurantii Immaturus) and Hou Po(Cortex Magnolia Officinalis) should be used first to dissipate stagnation of qi and accumulation of pathogenic factors, then, Wu Wei Yi Gong San (Miracle Powder of Five Drugs) plus Huo Xiang (Herba Agastachis) and Sha RN (Fructus Amomi) to reinforce qi of the middle-jiao. Overuse of drastic drugs with the action of relieving stagnation of qi should be avoided.

For the cases with regurgitation of food from the stomach one or half day after eating due to weakness of stomach qi with phlegm, Er Chen Tang(Two Old Drugs Decoction) plus RN Shen (Radix Ginseng), Bai Zhu (Rhizoma Atractylodis Macrocephalae), Huo Xiang (Herba Agastachis) and Ji Nei Jin (Endothelium Corneum Gigeriae Galli) should be selected, in cases of extremely weakened constitution, Pao Jiang (Baked Ginger) and Fu Zi (Radix Aconiti Praeparata) should be added.

Vomiting right after eating due to heat should be treated with the decoction of Bai Mao gen(Rhizoma Imperatae) and Lu Gen (Rhizoma Phragmitis).

For a dying patient with regurgitation and lassitude, 30-60 g of ginseng is to be decocted and taken with Ginger juice after the decoction is concentrated.

For the cases with weakened Mingmen fire failing to generate earch, Ba Wei

Di Huang Tang (Radix Rehmanniae Decoction Containing Eight Drugs) plus Ding Xiang (Flos Syzygii Aromatici) and Chen Xiang (Lignum Aquilariae Resinatum), or interval use of Hei Qian Dan (Bolus with Lead)is to be selected. They may also be treated with powder of Fu Zi (Radix Aconiti) by taking with saliva, 1. 5 to 3 g each time. (The powder was prepared as follows: dig a hole in a piece of Fu Zi with its tip removed, put 40g of Ding Xiang inside, then tie the tip and body of Fu Zi tightly to be decocted together with ginger juice and then ground into fine powder after baked). For cases with intense thirst, gruel porridge should be taken and foods greasy raw or cold should be avoided. For cases with extreme weakness, RN shen (Radix Ginseng) should be added.

For the cases with depletion of the stomach yin, the prescription selected is Xie Ding Yang Wei Tang (Acknowleged Decoction for Nourishing the Stomach), ingredients of which are:

Radix Adenophorae Strictae	15g
Radix Salivae Miltiorrhizae	15g
Poria	9g
Folium Eriobotryae	9g
Herba dendrobii	9g
Rhizoma Acori Graminei	9g
Caulis Bambusae in Taeniam	9g
Rhizoma Pinelliae	9g
Radix Glycyrrhizae	3g

Bamboo juice, Ginger jujce, Bei Mu (Bulbus Fritillariae), Gua Lou (Fructus Trichosanthis), RN Shen (Radix Ginseng), Mai Dong (Radix Opniopogonis), Tian Dong (Radix Asparagi), Bai Shao (Radix Paeoniae), Mu Gua (Fructus Chaenomelis), Wu Mei (Fructus Mume), and Suan Zao RN (Semen Ziziphi Spinocae) may be used as additional drugs.

For the cases with nausea, vomiting. anorexia, or vomiting right after eating due to the upward adverse flow of the liver-qi, the selected prescription is modified Shen Zhe Pei Qi Tang (Ginseng and RN Ochre Decoction for supplementing Qi) ingredients of which are:

Radix Ginseng
Ochra Raematitum
Rhizoma Pinelliae

Radix Asparagi
Flos Inulae
Pruina Kaki
Radix Notoginseng

IV   TCM THERAPY COORDINATING
WITH MODERN MEDICINAL TREATMENT

1. Postoperative recuperation with TCM and western medicine: Due to the stress of surgery and injury to visceral organs the impairment of the function of internal organs, yields abdominal distension, constipation, bitter sensation in mouth, thickly coated tongue, anorexia, diarrhea, and dyspepsia. In addition to replacing fluid supporting symptomatic therapy, invigorating the spleen and regulating the flow of qi, removing the obstruction of the bowel and lowering the adverse flow of qi should be undertaken. The prescriptions adopted are as follows:

Jianpi Yiqi Decoction

Radix Codonopsis	15g
Poria	12g
Radix Glycyrrhizae	3g
Rhizoma Atractylodi Macrocephalae	12g
Radix Astragali	15g
Radix Aucklandiae	9g
Radix Glehniae	9g
Pericarpium Citri Reticulate	8g
Semen Trichosanthis	15g
Fructus Hordei Germinatus	15g
Fructus Setariae Germinata	15g
Massa Medicata Fermentata	9g

Add or substract drugs according to existing symptoms.

Each dose boiled 3 times, 1 dose per day. Feed the decoction into stomach through nasal intubation, then tie the outlet of tube for downflow of drugs. Begin 2 to 3 days after surgery and continue for 3 to 7 days or more. This reduces post-operative side reactions and accelerates rehabilitation.

Weichang Fuyuan Decoction

Radix Astragali	15g
Radix Pseudostellariae	10g
Caulis Perillae	10g
Fructus Aurantii	10g
Radix et Rhizoma Rhei	15g
Semen Rapheni Parched	20g
Radix Aucklandiae	10g
Semen Persicae	10g
Radix Paeoniae Rubra	15g
Herba Taraxaci	20g

Boil for preparing decoction. Taken in 3 or 4 units oral or nasal feeding, for 3 days following surgery. Should be stopped or the dosage decreased when defecation exceeds 3 times per day. This prescription is now made into a paste and can be taken conveniently diluted with water. It will accelerate the recovery of gastro-intestinal function.

2. Postoperative chemotherapy coordinated with TCM: When single medicine chemotherapy is used in treating SC, the effective rate is around 20%. Some reports reveal the maximum effective rate of combined chemotherapy can reach over 50%. After surgery, as patients recover, chemotherapy should begin within two weeks to inhibit and eliminate the residual carcinoma cells.

3. Combined application of TCM drugs and chemotherapy: Chemotherapeutic drugs can compromise the qi of the human body, but coordinating them with TCM can alleviate adverse reactions, increase the patient's response to chemotherapy and enhance its efficacy. The prescription for "Bushen Jianpi Decoction" formulated according to the author's clinical experience has produced good therapeutic effects.

Radix Codonopsis	15g
Rhizoma Atractylodis Macrocephalae	12g
Poria	12g
Radix Glycyrrhizae	3g
Radix Astragali	15g
Fructus Ligustici Lucidi	15g

Fructus Lycii	12g
Radix Rehmanniae Preparata	15g
Rhizoma Polygonati	12g
Semen Nelumbins	15g
Semen Euryales	15g
Rhizoma Dioscoreae	12g
Radix Pseudostellariae	12g

Add or subtract drugs according to the symptoms existed.

Boil three times, one dose per day, to be taken concurrently with chemotherapy.

V COMBINED TREATMENT OF CHEMOTHERAPY AND TCM FOR CASES WHEN NO SURGERY BEEN PERFORMED

This section applies to cases of SC not indicated for surgery or for those who for various reasons are inoperable. In addition to Bushen Jianpi decoction, the following two prescriptions can be selected, depending on the patient's condition.

1. Liwei Huajie Decoction: Indicated for cases without pyloric obstruction.

Radix Codonopsis	15g
Rhizoma Atractylodis Macrocephalae	12g
Poria	12g
Radix Glycyrrhizae	3g
Radix Astragali	15g
Radix Rehmanniae Preparata	15g
Rhizoam Polygonati	12g
Herba Solanii Lyrati	30g
Herba Oldenlandiae Diffusae	30g
Semen Euryales	15g
Fructus Jujube	15g
Radix Glehniae	6g
Fructus Lycii	10g
Calculi Caprinus	9g

Radix Notoginseng   10g
   (finely ground)   1.5g

Boil each dose three times, place powder of Radix Notoginseng into a thermos cup, pour hot decoction from the first boiling into the cup, stir until the powder is dissolved. Cover the cup for 5 to 10 minutes, then take the drug orally. Do not add more Radix Notoginseng to the second and third boiled decoctions.

2. Liwei Tongguan Decoction: Indicated for cases complicated by pyloric obstruction, belching with fetid odor as well as acid regurgitation. In addition to the above prescription of Liwei Huajie Decoction, add Flos Inulae 9g, Haematitum 12g, Rhizoma Pinelliae 6g, Fructus Evodiae (prepared with Rhizoma Coptidis) 6g, Fructus Hordei Germinatus 15g and subtract Radix Rehmanniae Preparata, Rhizoma Polygonati, Fructus Jujube and Fructus Lycii.

Mothod of adding or subtracting drugs for these two recipes according to symdrome differentiation:

Asthenia cold of stomach and spleen: Add Fructus Amomi, Fructus Amomi Rotundus, Radix Aconiti Lateralis Preparata, increase the amount of Radix Notoginseng, reduce the amount of Herba Solanii Lyrati, Radix Glehniae and Herba Oldenlandiae Difffusae.

Consumption of yin by stomach-heat manifested as dry mouth and red crimson tongue: Add Radix Ophiopogonis, Rhizoma Polygonati Odorati, Rhizoma Anemarrhenae, Herba Dendrobii, Radix Asparagi, exchange Radix Codonopsis for Radix Pseudostellariae, reduce the amount of Radix Rehmanniae Preparata, Fructus Jujube and Radix Notoginseng.

Asthenia of qi and blood, Expressed as leukopenia: Add Caulis Spatholobi, Fructus Ligustici Lucidi, Radix Angelicae sinensis, increase amount of Radix Astragali.

Hematemesis and hematochezia: Add Folium Callicarpae Pedunculatae, Herba Agrimoniae, Flos Lonicerae, Crinis Carbonisatus, Colla Corii Asini and Bletiliae fructus.

Constipation: Add Fructus Trichosanthis, Fructus Cannabis, Radix et Rhizoma Rhei, Herba Cistanches, Folium Sennae. Reduce amount of Fructus Jujube, Radix Notoginseng and Radix Rehmanniae Preparata.

Diarrhea: Add Pericarpium Papaveris, Cortex Fraxini, Cortex Magnoliae

Officinalis, Rhizoma Coptidis and Herba Chelidonii. Reduce amount of Herba Oldenlandiae Diffusae and Herba Solanii Lyrati.

Anorexia: Add Fructus Setariae Geriminatus, Fructus Hordei Germinatus, Fructus Crataegi Ebdothelium, Corneum Gigenae Galli and Massa Medicata Fermentata. Reduce amount of Radix rehmanniae Prepatata and Fructus Jujube. Pain: Rhizoma Corydalis and Radix Linderae are added.

Edema: Semen Plantaginis, Poria, Polyporus and Radix Alismatis are added.

VI TCM THERAPY COORDINATING WITH RADIOTHERAPY

Liwei Huajie Decoction, with addition or subtraction of drugs depending on the syndrome differentiation, is used as adjuvant therapy. If the asthenia of yin and yang or disturbance of gastrointestinal function appears, the following prescription is used:

Radix Ophiopogonis	12g
Radix Glehniae	10g
Rhizoma Polygonati Odorati	9g
Poria	12g
Rhizoma Atractylodis Macrocephalae	10g
Radix Codonopsis	12g
Radix Glycyrrhizae	3g
Endothelium Corneum Gigeriae Galli	9g
Massa Medicata Fermentata	9g
Radix Astragali	15g
Radix Pseudostellariae	12g

Decoct each dose 3 times, 1 dose per day, taken orally in three equal portions.

Chapter Sixteen

Recipes for Treating Disorders of Digestive System

Aconite bolus for Regulating the function of Meddle-jiao
(Fu zi li zhong wan)

INGREDIENTS

Radix Aconiti Lateralis Praeparata

Radix Codonopsis Pilosulae

Rhizoma Atractylodis Mocrocephalae

Rhizoma Zingiberis

Radix Glycyrrhizae

Honeyed boluses, 9g each bolus, 10 boluses per box.

INDICATIONS

Warming the middle-jiao and invigorating the spleen. Insufficiency of yang in the spleen and stomach, manifested as abdominal cold-pain, vomiting, diarrhea and cold limbs.

DIRECTION

To be taken orally, 1 bolus each time, 2-3 times a day.

Aucklandia-coptis Pill
(Xing lian wan)

INGREDIENTS

Rhizoma Coptidis

Radix Aucklandiae

Water-honeyed pills, 18g per bottle.

ACTIONS

Clearing away pathogenic heat and dampness, promoting the circulation of qi and removing obstruction.

INDICATIONS

Dysentery due to damp-heat pathogen, manifested as abdominal pain, diarrhea, pus and blood in the stool, and tenesmus. It can be used for bacillary dysentery and enteritis.

DIRECTION To

be taken orally, 3-6g each time, twice a day. For children, the doses should be correspondingly reduced.

Bolus Containing Five Seeds
(Wu ren wan)

INGREDIENTS

Semen Biota	3. 8g
Semen Persicae	15g
Semen Armeniacae Amarum	30g
Semen Pini	3g
Semen Pruni	3g
Pericarpium Citri Reticulatae	120g

INDICATIONS

Lubricating intestines and promoting bowel movement. It is indicated for constipation attributive to dryness of intestines, since it is composed chiefly of fatty seeds.

Bolus for Regulating the
function of Middle-warmer
(Li zhong wan)

INGREDIENTS

Radix Ginseng	90g
Rhizoma Zingiberis	90g
Rhizoma Atractylodis Macrocephalae	90g
Radix Glycyrrhizae Praeparata	90g

Grind the above drugs and make them into boluses, take the boluses orally with warm boiled water, 9g each time, two or three times a day.

INDICATIONS

Warming the middle-warmer to dispel cold replenishing qi to invigorate the spleen. Hypofunction of the spleen and stomach marked by abdominal pain with predilection for warmth and for pressure by hand, watery diarrhea, fullness of the abdomen, anorexia, vomiting, pale tongue with white coating, deep and thready pulse; or manifested by bleeding due to yang-deficiency; or chronic infantile convulsion.

The recipe can be modified to treat cold syndromes due to hypofunction of the spleen and stomach as seen in cases of chronic gastritis, gastroduodenal ulcer, chronic colitis, indigestion, gastric dilatation, gastropotosia, or cold syndromes of excess type in the spleen and stomach as seen in cases of acute gastritis and enteritis.

Since the recipe tends to be warm and dry in property, it is not advisable for cases with fever due to exopathogens, or with internal heat due to yin deficiency.

INTERPRETATION

Of the ingredients in the recipe, Dried ginger, with its pungent hot property attributing to the channels of the spleen and stomach, acts as a principal drug and is to restore the yang of the spleen and somach by means of warming the middle-warmer to dispel cold, to arrest vomiting by way of regulating the stomach to send down reversed flow of qi. Ginseng, slightly bitter in flavor and slightly warm in nature, is administered as an assistant drug for tonifying qi, strengthening the spleen and stomach. Bighead atractylodes rhizome, with its sweet and bitter flavour and warm nature attributing to the channel of spleen, serves as an adjuvant drug for strengthening the spleen and eliminating dampness. Prepared licorice root, sweet and mild in property, attributing to the channel of spleen, replenishes the spleen-qi and regulates the middle-warmer, and tempers the effect of other drugs in the recipe, playing the part of a guiding drug.

Modern researches have ascertained that this recipe has the afficacies in adjusting the functions of the stomach and intestine, promoting blood circulation, strengthening metabolism, relieving spasm, alleviating pain, arresting vomiting and diarrhea, inducing diuresis, etc.

Chidren's Dysentery Tablet
(Xiao er xie li pain)

INGREDIENTS (Omitted)

ACTIONS

Clearing away pathogenic heat and dampness, arresting diarrhea and treating dysentery.

INDICATIONS

Diarrhea due to pathogenic dampness and heat, dysentery with bloody or mucous stool.

DIRECTION

To be taken orally, children: under one yeay old, 1 tablet; 1-2 years old, 1-2 tablets; 2-4 years old, 2-3 tablets; 4-7 years old, 3-4 tablets; 7-14 years old, 4-6 tablets each time. All 4 times a day.

Tablets, each tablet equals 0.5g crude drug.

Children's Indigestion Tablet
(Xiao er xiao shi pain)

INGREDIENTS

Endothelium Corneum Gigeriae Galli

Fructus Crataegi

Massa Fermentata Medicinalis

Fructus Hordei Germinatus

Semen Arecae

Pericarpium Citri Reticulatae

Tablets, 0.3 g each tablet.

ACTIONS

Strengthening the spleen, regulating the stomach, promoting digestion and eliminating indigested food.

INDICATIONS

Incoordination between the spleen and the stomach, indigestion, poor appetite, abdominal distension, constipation; retention of food in the stomach, malnutrition, etc.

DIRECTION

To be taken orally, children 1-3 years old: 2-4 tablets; 3-7 years old: 4-6 tablets each time, all 3 times a day. Adults: 6-8 tablets each time, 3 times a day.

Compound Hepatitis-treating Infusion
(Fu fang gan yan chong ji)

INGREDIENTS

Radix Bupleuri

Herba Artemisiae Capillaris

Radix Glycyrrhizae

Herba Hyperici Japonici

Herba Taraxaci

Herba Lysimachiae

Medicinal granules (infusion), 14g each packet, 10 packets per box.

ACTIONS

Clearing wawy heat, dispersing the depressed liver-qi normalizing the functioning of gallbladder.

INDICATIONS

Acute icterohepatitis, acute non-icterohepatitis, hepatitis of persisting type and cholocystitis.

DIRECTION

To be taken orally after being infused in warm boiled water, 1 packet each time, twice a day.

Compound Oral Liquid of Isatis Leaf
(Fu fang da qing ye he ji)

INGREDIENTS

Folium Isatidis

Flos Lonicerae

Rhizoma seu Radix Notopterygii

Rhizoma Bistortae

Radix et Rhizoma Rhei

Oral liquid, 10ml per bottle, and 100ml per bottle.

ACTIONS

Clearing away pestilence and toxic materials.

INDICATIONS

Influenza, upper respiratory tract infection, acute and chronic hepatitis, parotitis, etc.

DIRECTION

To be taken orally 10-15ml each time, 2-3 times a day. The dosage for children should be reduced accordingly.

Decoction Containing Three Kinds of Seed for the Aged
(San zi yang qin tang)

INGREDIENTS

Semen Sinapis Albae	10g
Fructus Perillae	12g
Semen Raphani	15g

ACTION

Lowering the adverse rising energy, promoting digestion, warming and dispersing phlegm; mainly for the aged with hypofunciton of the spleen and stagnation of phlegm and vital energy, manifested as cough with profuse expectoration, dyspnea, feeling of oppression over the chest, anorexia, white and greasy fur on the tongue, smooth pulse, etc.

INDICATIONS

1. For those cases with profuse expectoration of thin sputum, which are attributive to retention of cold-phlegm in the lung, add Rhizoma Zingiberis. For those with feeling of oppression over the chest, shortness of breath, difficult expectoration, which are attributive to stagnation of vital energy by phlegm, add Semen Armeniacae Amarum and Cortex Magnoliae Officinalis.

2. Applicable to cases of hiccup accompanied with profuse expectoration,

feeling of oppression over the chest, white and greasy fur on the tongue, wiry and smooth pulse, which are attributive to stagnation of phlegm and vital energy and dysfunction of stomach.

3. Also applicable to cases of senile emphysema, chronic bronchitis, gastritis, duodenal ulcer, etc., marked by cough and hiccup, which are attributive to stagnation of vital energy and phlegm.

INTERPRETATION

All the three drugs used in the prescription are expectorants. Sinapis is superior for waming lung and benefiting vital energy, and should be used as the principal drug for the cases with chest fullness and profuse expectoration. Perillae is superior for lowering the adverse rising energy and relieving dyspnea, and should be used as the principal drug for cases with dyspneic cough. Raphani is superior for promoting digestion, and should be used as a chief drug fro cases with anorexia. But this prescription exerts a sinking (lowering)action, and just serves as a symptomatic remedy. As soon as the symptoms subside, a therapy of invigorating middle-jiao energy should be applied.

Decoction for Invigorating
the Spleen and Nourishing the Heart (1)
(Gui pi tang)

SOURCE Recipes for Saving Lives

INGREDIENTS

Radix Astragali Seu Hedysari	15g
Radix Codonopsis Pilosulae	15g
Radix Angelicae Sinensis	12g
Arillus Longan	12g
Rhizoma Atractylodis Macrocephalae	10g
Poria	10g
Semen Ziziphi Spinosae	10g
Radix Aucklandiae	5g
Radix Glycyrrhizae Praeparata	5g
Radix Polysalae	3g

| Rhizoma Zingiberis Recens | 5 pcs |
| Fructus Ziziphi Jujubae | 5 pcs |

INDICATIONS

Benefiting vital enerty, strengthening spleen, invigorating the heart and nourishing blood; mainly for cases due to hypofunction of heart and spleen and insufficiency of vital energy and blood manifested as pal-pitation, amnesia, insomnia, fatigue, poor appetite, sallow complexion, or preceded menstrual cycle with profuse pale or continuously dripping discharge, pale tongue with whitish fur, small and weak pulse.

For cases of metrorrhagia attributive to failure of the spleen to control blood, subtract Aucklandiae and polygalae and add Fructus Corni to nourish liver and stop metrorrhagia. For cases with bloody stools affributive to hypofunction of spleen with retention of cold evil, substract Polygalae and add Zingiberis Praeparata to warm middle jiao and stopping bleeding.

Also applicable to cases of peptic ulcer, dysfunctional uterine bleeding, thrombocytopeina purpura, aplastic anemia, etc. with hemorrhage attributive to hypofunction of heart and spleen.

INTERPRETATION

Astragali seu Hedysari and Codonopsis Pilosulae benefit vital energy and invigorate the spleen and serve as the chief drugs. Angelicae Sinensis and Arillus Longan tonify the blood, nourish the heart. The above four drugs used together strengthen both the heart and the spleen, and dealt with the primary aspect of the disease. Poria, Polygalae, Ziziphi Spinosae have the effects of nourishing the heart and calming the mental state, and dealt with the secondary aspect of the disease. Aucklandiae and Atractylodis Macrocephalae strengthen the spleen and regulate vital energy. Glycyrrhizae, Zingiberis recens and Ziziphi Jujubae reconcile the action of spleen and stomach, and promote the production of vital energy and blood. In summary, this prescription aims at benefiting vital energy and tonifying blood, when one's vital energy is sufficient, the heart is well nourished, the symptoms subside.

Decoction for Invigorating
the Spleen and Nourishing the Heart (2)
(Gui pi tang)

SOURCE Prescriptions for Succouring the Sick

INGREDIENTS

Rhizoma Atractylodis Macrocephalae	30g
Poria cum Ligno Hospite	30g
Radix Astragali seu Hedysari	30g
Arillus Longan	30g
Semen Ziziphi spinosae (stir-fried, shell removed)	30g
Radix Ginseng	15g
Radix Aucklandiae	15g
Radix Glycyrrhizae Preaparata	8g
Radix Angelicae Sinensis	3g
Radix Polygalae (honey-parched)	3g

With the addition of fresh ginger 6g and Chinese-dates 3-5 pcs. , all the drugs are decocted in water for oral administration.

INDICATIONS

Replenishing qi and tonifying the blood, invigorating the spleen and nourishing the heart.

Weakness of both the spleen and heart marked by palpitation or severe palpitation, amnesia, insomnia, night sweat, fever of deficient type, anorexia, general debility, sallow complexion, pale tongue with thin and whitish coating, and thready and loose pulse; hemafecia due to dysfuncton of the spleen in governing the blood, metrorrhagia, metrostaxis, preceded menstrual period with excessive blood loss in light colour,. and continuous dripping of menstruation or morbid leukorrhagia, etc.

Moreover, the recipe can be modified to treat other cases such as disturbance of the vegetative nerve, menopausal syndrome, cardiac neurosis, insomnia, amnesia, anemia, thrombocytopenia, hypoproteinemia, chronic gastroenteritis, nervous gastritis, uterine functional bleeding that are ascribed to insufficiency of both the spleen and heart.

The recipe should not be administered to those with heat-evil hidden interiorly and those with rapid pulse due to yin deficiency.

INTERPRETATION

In the recipe, astragalus root and ginseng as principal drugs, have the effects of tonifying qi and invigorating the spleen; bighead atractylodes rhizoma and Prepared licorice root assist the principal drugs in reinforcing the spleen and replenishing qi. Chinese angelica root is good at enriching the liver to promote the generation of heart-blood; Nos. 2, 4 and 5, function in nourishing the heart and tranquilizing the mind; Polygala root has the effect of relieving mental stress; Aucklandia root has the effect of regulating the flow of qi and enlivening the spleen and is used to prevent qi-replenishing drugs and blood tonics from causing stagnation of qi and interfering the functions of the spleen and stomach.

Recent studies have proved that this recipe is effective for promoting digestion and absorption, strengthening metabolism, consolidating the constitution by nourishing the body, regulating the excitement of the cerebrum, promoting gastrointestinal peristalsis as well as arresting diarrhia.

Decoction for Lifting Yang-Energy
and Benefiting stomach
(Sheng yang yi wei tang)

INGREDIENTS

Radix Astragali seu Hedysari	12g
Radix Codonopsis Pilosulae	10g
Radix Paeoniae Alba	10g
Rhizoma Atractylodis Macrocephalae	10g
Poria	10g
Rhizoma Pinelliae	6g
Rhizoma et Radix Notopterygii	6g
Radix Angelicae Pubescentis	6g
Radix Ledebouriellae	6g
Exocarpium Citri Grandis	6g
Rhizoma Alismatis	6g

Radix Bupleuri	6g
Radix Glycyrrhizae Praeparata	3g
Rhizoma Coptidis	3g
Rhizoma Zingiberis Recens	5 Pcs
Fructus Ziziphi Jujubae	3 Pcs

All the above drugs are decocted in water for oral administration.

ACTION

Lifting yang-energy, invigorating the spleen, benefiting the stomach, expellling wind and dampness; mainly for cases attributive to hypofunction of the spleen and stomach and stagnation of dampness, which manifest as general aching, fatigue, poor appetite, chilliness, bitter taste in the mouth, dry tongue, frequent urination, pale and corpulent tongue, white and smooth fur, slow and soft, floating pulse.

INDICATIONS

1. Indicated for cases attributive to deficiency of spleen-energy and stomach-energy and the attack of exogenous wind-dampness, which manifest as chilliness, sweating, soreness of limbs, tiredness, stuffy nose with nasal discharge, pale tongue with thin and white fur, floating and large or floating and slow pulse.

2. Applicable to cases with lienteric diarrhea, increased borborygmus abdominal fullness, anorexia, epigastric upset after meal, spiritlessness, fatigue, pale tongue with white and smooth fur, slow and soft, floating pulse, which are attributive to hypofunction of spleen and accumulation of dampness in the stomach and intestines.

3. Also applicable to cases of pulmonary tuberculosis, chronic cholecystitis, emphysema complicated by pulmonary infection, chronic gastroenteritis, pancreatitis irritable colon, which are attributive to hypofunction of spleen and accumulation of dampness.

INTERPRETATION

Codonopsis Pilosulae, Atractylodis Macrocephalae, Poria, Glycyrrhizae Praeparata, Citri Grandis, Pinelliae and Astragali seu Hedysari can invigorate middle jiao , benefite vital energy, promote the function of spleen and dry dampness. Codonopsis Pilosulae and Astragali seu Hedysari also have a strong effect on invigorating the lung and the spleen, and benefiting vital energy and wei-energy. Bupleuri, Ledebouriellae, Notopterygii and Angelicae Pubescentis serve to lift up yang-energy and eliminate wind and dampness when used together with Astragali seu Hedysari. Alismatis used together with Poria can promote diuresis to relieve frequent micturition resulting from dysfunction of spleen. Coptidis serves as a stomachic to improve the digestive function. Zingiberis and Ziziphi Jujuba are applied for regulating ying and wei and help the above drugs to support healthy energy and eliminate evils.

Decoction for Mildly Warming the Middle Jiao
(Xiao jian zhong tang)

INGREDIENTS

Ramulus Cinnamomi	10g
Radix Paeoniae Alba	20g
Rhizoma Zingiberis Recens	6 Pcs
Radix Glycyrrhizae Praeparata	6g
Fructus Ziziphi Jujubae	8 Pcs
Saccharum Granorum	30g

All the above drugs are decocted in water for oral administration.

ACTION

Waming middle jiao, tonifying energy, regulating the interior and relieving the acute condition; mainly for cases due to asthenia-cold of middle jiao and dysfunction of liver and spleen, manifested as abdominal pain which can be relieved by warmth and pressure.

INDICATIONS

1. By adding Radix Angelicae Sinensis, another prescription named Decoction with Angelicae Sinensis for Mildly Warming the Middle Jiao (from Supplement to Valuable Prescriptions) is formed. It has the effects of regulating ying promoting blood circulation, relieving pain and acute condition, and is indicated for cases of postpartum abdominal pain attributed to deficiency of ying-blood.

2. By adding Radix Astragali seu Hedysari, another prescription named Decoction with Astragali seu Hedysari, for Mildly Warming the Middle Jiao (from Synopsis of Golden Cabinet) is formed. It has the effects of arresting abnormal

sweating and strengthening superficial resistance, regulating and invigorating yin and yang, and is indicated for cases of spontaneous sweating and shortness of breath attributed to imbalance between yin and yang and disorders of vital energy and blood.

3. Applicable to the cases of fever caused by the deficiency of vital energy or imbalance between yin and yang and disorders of vital energy and blood.

4. Also applicable to the cases of gastroduodenal ulcer, gastritis and pancreatitis with abdominal pain attributed to asthenia-cold of middle jiao, and cases of functional fever and aplastic anemia with fever attributed to imbalance between yin and yang and disorders of vital energy and blood.

INTERPRETATION

Saccharum Granorum, sweet in taste and slightly warm in nature, has the effects of tonifying, strengthening middle jiso, invigorating both spleen-yin and spleen-yang , but its analgesic effect is relatively mild; Ramulus Cinnamomi, acrid and sweet in taste and warm in nature, has a stronger effects of warming yang-energy and eliminating cold evil and relieving pain, although its tonifying effect is milder but its analgesic effect is stronger. The two drugs used together act as the principal remedy fro severe abdominal pain of asthenia-cold type. Paeoniae Alba is applied with a double dosage of Ramulus Cinnamomi, and helps Glycyrrhizae and saccharum Granorum to soften the liver and relieve pain. Zingiberis Reccens, Ziziphi Jujubae and Glycyrrhizae Praeparata used together aim at strengthening spleen-yang.

Decoction for Mild Phlegm-heat
Syndrome in the Chest
(Xiao xian xiong tang)

INGREDIENTS

Rhizoma Copitdis	10g
Rhizoma Pinelliae (washed)	10g
Fructus Trichosanthis	25g

All the above drugs are decocted in water for oral administration.

ACTION

Clearing away heat evil, eliminating phlegm, soothing the chest and dispersing stagnation; mainly for mild syndrome of phlegm-heat stagnation in the thorax, which is manifested as feeling of oppression over the chest with pain and tenderness, cough with yellow and thick sputum, and greasy fur on the tongue, floating and smooth or rapid and somooth pulse.

INDICATIONS

1. Applicable to cases with abdominal fullness, tenderness, nausea, vomiting, expectoration of yellow and thick sputum, are attributive to stagnation of phlegm and heat or dampness-heat in the middle jiao (stomach and gallbladder).

2. Also applicable to cases of exudative pleuritis, bronchitis, pneumonia, etc., marked by feeling of oppression over the chest and tenderness, or acte gastritis, cholecystitis, viral hepatitis, etc., marked by fullness over the epigastrium and lypochondrium and tenderness, wich are attributive to the stagnation of phlegm and heat.

INTERPRETATION

Trichosanthis has the effects of clearing away heat evil, eliminating phlegm, soothing the chest and dispersing stagnation, and serves as the chief drug used in large dosage; Pinelliae is applied to eliminate phlegm and disperse stagnation, and Coptidis to clear away heat evil and inhibit fire. The two drugs act together to relieve the stagnation of phlegm and heat evil and lower the abnormal rising enegry and heat evil in the chest.

Decoction for Reinforcing the Viscera
(Zhen ren yang zang tang)

INGREDIENTS

Radix Ginseng	6g
Radix Angelicae Sinensis	9g
Rhizoma Atractylodis Macrocephalae	12g
Semen Myristicae	12g
Cortex Cinnamomi	3g
Radix Glycyrrhizae Praeparata	6g
Radix Paeoniae Alba	15g

Radix Aucklandiae	9g
Fructus Chebulae	12g
Pericarpium Papaveris	20g

All the drugs should be decocted in water for oral administration.

INDICATIONS

Warming and tonifying the spleen-yang to arrest diarrhea.

Chronic diarrhea or chronic dysentery due to deficiency and coldness of the spleen and kidney manifested as prolonged diarrhea or dysentery, incontinence of the feces due to lingering diarrhea or prolapse of anus which fails to be elevated again, abdominal pain that may be relieved by warmness and pressure, listlessness, poor appetite, pale tongue with whitish fur, and deep and slow pulse.

Chronic enteritis, intestinal tuberculosis, chronic dysentery, prolapse of rectum and other diseases marked by lingering diarrhea due to deficiency of yang can be treated by the modified recipe.

The recipe is contraindicated in patients with primary symptoms of dysentery still with accumulation of toxic heat.

INTERPRETATION

Poppy capsule used in large dosage, relieves diarrhea with astringency, and bark of Chinese cassia tree warms the kidney and spleen, both acting as principal drugs. As assistant drugs, Nutmeg warms the kidney and spleen to act on the intestine with its astringency; Myrobalan arrests diarrhea with its astringency; Ginseng and Bighead atractylodes rhizome invigorate qi and strengthen the spleen. Chinese angelica root and White peong root enrich the blood and regulate ying, and Aucklandia root regulates qi to remove stagnancy and arrest pain, acting as asjuvant drugs together. Prepared licorice root coordinates the effectes of the other drugs in the recipe and regulate the stomach, combined with white peony root it can relieve spasm to arrest pain as a guiding drug.

Modern researches have proved that the recipe has the effects of strengthening the human body, regulating the gastrointestinal peristalsis, relieving spasm, promoting blood circulation and relieving diarrhea.

Decoction for Warming Spleen
(Wen pi tang)

INGREDIENTS

Radix Aconiti Praeparata	10g
Radix et Rhizoma Rhei (decocted later)	10g
Radix Codonopsis Pilosulae	10g
Rhizoma Zingiberis (dried)	6g
Radix Glycyrrhizae	3g

ACTION

Warming the interior to promote the bowel movement, regulating and invigorating spleen-yang; mainly for cases with constipation or chronic diarrhea due to insufficiency of spleen -yang and accumulation of cold evil in the interior, which are manifested with abdominal pain with desire for warmth, cold limbs, whitish and greasy fur on the tongue, sunken and wiry pulse.

INDICATION

1. For cases of chronic dysentery with grey and greasy fur on the tongue signifying a more severe retention of cold evil, subtract Codonopsis Pilosulae and Glycyrrhizae and add Cortex Cinnamomi, Radix Angelicae Sinensis to expel cold and regulate blood.

2. Also applicable to cases of gastrolithiasis, chronic bacillary dysentery, amebic dysentery, chronic colitis, etc. with constipation or diarrhea, which are attributive to asthenia-syndrome complicated by sthenia-syndrome.

3. Decoction of Rhei and Aconiti Praeparata and this prescription both have the effects of warming the interior and promoting bowel movement, and are applicabe for constipation with retention of cold evil. The former is more suitable for the cases when the evil is hyperactive and the healthy energy is not yet deficient, while the latter one is suitable for those when the healthy energy is already deficient (insufficiency of spleen-yang).

INTERPRETATION

Rhei, bitter in taste and cold in nature, is a strong purgative which should not be used alone for cases with insufficiency of spleen-yang. In this prescription, Aconiti which has a strong action for warming spleen and expelling cold is used simultaneously, and an effect of warming the interior and promoting bowel movement is obtained. Zingiberis, Codonopsis Pilosulae, Glycyrrhizae can enhance the effects of Aconiti for warming and invigorating yang-energy. All the above drugs used together serve as an ideal formula for warming spleen to promote bowel movement.

Decoction of Artemisiae Annuae and Scutellariae
for Clearing Away Dampness-heat in Gallbladder
(Hao qin qing dan tang)

INGREDIENTS

Herba Artemisiae Annuae	10g
Radix Scutellariae	10g
Poria	10g
Caulis Bambusae in Taeniam	10g
Rhizoma Pinelliae Praeparata	6g
Fructus Aurantii	6g
Exocarpium Citri Grandis	6g
Green Jade Powder (Six to One Powder with Indigo Naturalis)	10g

ACTION

Clearing away the heat evil in gallbladder, eliminating dampness evil and phlegm; mainly for cases due to stagnation of dampness and heat evil in the gallbladder, which are manifested as alternating episodes of chills and fever (more prominent), distending pain of the upper abdomen, bitter taste in the mouth, acid or bile regurgitation, red tongue with yellowish and greasy fur, wiry and rapid pulse.

INDICATION

1. For cases with vomiting, add Zuojin Bolus (Rhizoma Coptidis and Fructus Evodiae) to clear away heat evil in the liver and gallbladder, lower the abnormal rising energy and stop vomiting; for cases with whitish and greasy fur, smooth and rapid pulse, attributive to severe affection of dampness and heat evil, omit glycyrrhizae and add fructus Tsaoko or Fructus Amomi Cardamomi to dis-

perse the dampness evil.

2. For cases of jaundice with infreguent mictorition of yellow urine, attributive to severe affection of heat than dampness, omit Citri Grandis, Pinelliae Praeparata and glycyrrhizae and add Herba Artemisiae Scopariae to clear away heat evil, promote diuresis and relieve jaundice..

3. Also applicable to cases of cholecystitis, pancreatitis, gastritis, acute infectious icterus hepatitis, etc., which are attributive to stagnation of dampness-heat in the gallbladder.

INTERPRETATION

This prescription is composed by adding Artemisiae Annuae, Scutellariae, Talcum and Indigo Naturalis to Decoction for Clearing Away Gallbladder Heat. Artemisiae, Scutellariae and Indigo Naturalis have the effect of clearing away the gallbladder heat. Moreover Decoction for Clearing Away Gallbaladder Heat has the effects of drying the dampness and eliminating phlegm. Talcum has the effects of clearing away heat evil and promoting diuresis, letting the dampness-heat evil out from the urine. All the above drugs use together can clear away heat evil, promote the secretion of bile, eliminating dampness and phlegm, thus the disorder of gallbladder and stomach would be relieved and symptoms subsided.

Decoction of Astragali seu Hedysari for Warming Millde Jiao (Huang qi jian zhong tang)

INGREDIENT

Ramulus Cinnamomi	10g
Rhizoma Zingiberis Recens	10g
Radix Paeonie Alba	20g
Radix Astragali seu Hedysari	15g
Radix Glycyrrhizae Praeparata	6g
Saccharum Granorum	30g
Fructus Ziziphi Jujubae	7 Pcs

ACTION

Warming middle jiao, tonifying, alleviating pain, harmonizing yin and yang, and regulating ying and wei; mainly for consumptive diseases attributive

· 177 ·

to insufficiency of yin and yang (mainly deficiency of spleen-yang), which manifest as abdominal pain that can be alleviated by warmth and pressure, spontaneous sweating, shortness of breath, pale complexion, pale and corpulent tongue with whitish fur, large and weak pulse.

INDICATION

1. Applicable to cases of fever attributive to deficiency of spleen- and stomach-energy, and floating up of yang-energy, which manifest as increase of body temperature with preference for hot drink, aversion to cold, cold limbs, sweating, shortness of breath, fatigue, poor appetite, pale tongue with white fur, floating and large weak pulse.

2. Also indicated for cases of jaundice attributive to hypofunction of spleen, decreased production of vital energy and blood, and failure of nourishing skin and muscles, which manifest as yellowish coloration, dryness and lusterless appearance of the skin, shortness of breath, fatigue, polyuria with clear urine, pale and swelling tongue, white and smooth fur, slow pulse.

3. Also applicable to cases of gastroptosis, peptic ulcer, prolapse of gastric mucosa, leukemia, aplastic anemia, pulmonary tuberculosis, hemolytic jaundice, ancylostomiasis, etc. attributive to hypofunction of spleen.

INTERPRETATION

This prescription is formed by adding Astragali seu Hedysari to the Decoction for Mildly Warming Middle Jiao, which is used for warming middle jiao to relieve pain. Astragali seu Hedysari can warm spleen-yang when it combines with Ramulus Cinnamomi and Saccharum Granorum, can activate spleen-yang to increase the production of blood and vital energy when it combines with Zingiberis Recens and Ziziphi Jujubae, and also can benefit vital energy and strengthen yin to invigorate the superficies and stop sweating when it combines with Paeoniae Alba. In sum, this prescription is suitable for cases with deficiency of yin and yang resulting from hypofunction of spleen and stomach, and decreased production of vital energy and blood.

Decoction of Baked Yellow Earth
(Huang tu tang)

INGREDIENTS

Terra Flava Vsta	30g
Rhizoma Atractylodis Macrocephalae	9g
Radix Aconite Praeparata	9g
Radix Rehmanniae	9g
Colla Corii Asini	9g
Radix Scutellariae	9g
Radix Glycyrrhizae	9g

Decoct the baked yellow earth in water to get its decoction and then decoct the other drugs in the decoction for oral administration.

INDICATIONS

Warming yang, strengthening the spleen, nourishing the blood and stopping bleeding.

Hemorrhage which belongs to cold syndrome of insufficiency type manifested by hematemesis, epistaxis, hematochezia and metrorrhagia characterized by dark-red blood, cold limbs, sallow complexion, pale tongue with white fur, and deep thready and feeble pulse.

Patients with chronic hemorrhage of gastrointestinal tract and chronic dysfunctional uterine bleeding, marked by the symptoms of cold syndrome of insufficiency type can be treated by the modified recipe.

Patients with symptoms due to exogenous pathogenic factors should not be treated by this recipe.

INTERPRETATION

Baked yellow earth as a principal drug in the recipe, warms the middle-warmer to stop bleeding. Large-headed atractylodes rhizome and Prepared aconite root warm yang and strengthen the spleen and plays the role of assistant drugs. Dried rehmannia root and Donkey-hide gelatin nourish yin, supplement the blood and stop bleeding, thus not only helping baked yellow earth in stopping bleeding but also compensating for the loss of yin-blood. Scutellaria root bitter in taste and cold in nature, can be used together with Dried rehmannia root and

Donkey-hide gelatin to restrict the pungent, warm, dry and drastic nature of No. 2 and No. 3 to prevent wasting the blood. The drugs from No. 4 and No. 6 are adjuvent drugs. Licorice root as a guiding drugs coordinates the actions of the other drugs in the recipe and regulates the middle-warmer.

Modern researches have proved that the recipe can produce the effects of protecting the gastrointestinal mucous membrane, promoting the healing of ulcers, shortening the clotting time, promoting the regeneration of red blood cells and increasing hemoglobin.

Decociton of Caryophylli and Calyx Kaki
(Ding xiang shi ti tang)

INGREDIENTS

Flos Caryophylli	10g
Calyx Kaki	10g
Radix Codonopsis Pilosulae	6g
Rhizoma Zingiberis Recens	12g

INDICATIONS

Lowering the adverse rising of gas, relieving hiccup, warming middle jiao and benefiting vital energy; mainly for cases with asthenia-cold of stomach-energy, manifested as hiccup, pale tongue with whitish fur, sunken and slow pulse.

This is a prescription usually applied for cases of hiccup due to stomach-cold. For cases accompanied with stagnation of vital energy and phlegm, add Lignum Aquilariae Resinatum and Rhizoma Pinelliae Praeparata to regulate vital energy and disperse phlegm, also to enhance the effects of warming middle jiao and lowering the adverse rising of gas.

Also applicable to cases of nervous hiccup and hiccup after abdominal operation which are attributive to asthenia-cold of stomach-enegy.

INTERPRETATION

Caryophylli is acrid in taste and warm in nature, and has the effects of warming the stomach and relieving hiccup. Calyx Kaki and Zingiberis Recens enhance the effect of Caryophylli. Codonopsis Pilosulae has the effect of strengthening the spleen and stomach, it acts with caryophylli to regulate the ascending-descending function of stomach-energy, and both of them constituent an important pain for hiccup of spleen-hypofunction type. This is a representative prescription which dealts with both the principal and secondary problems, i. e., warming the spleen and stomach as well as relieving hiccup.

Decoction of Citri Grandis
(Da ju pi tang)

INGREDIENTS

Poria	10g
Polyporus Umbellatus	10g
Rhizoma Alismatis	10g
Rhizoma Atractylodis Macrocephalae	10g
Semen Arecae	10g
Cortex Cinnamomi	2g
Talcum	18g
Exocarpium Citri Grandis	6g
Radix Aucklandiae	6g
Radix Glycyrrhizae	3g
Rhizoma Zingiberis Recens	5Pcs

All the above drugs are decocted in water for oral administration.

ACTION

Activating the circulation of vital energy, promoting diuresis and clearing away dampness-heat; mainly for cases attributive to impairment of vital energy by the combined attack of dampness and heat, which manifest as abdominal fullness and pain, watery diarrhea, extreme thirst, reddish urine, red tongue with yellow and greasy fur, soft and floating, rapid pulse.

INDICATION

Applicable to cases with pitted edema of the extremities, which are attributive to retention of dampness in the interior with formation of heat. Also applicable to cases attributive to the dysfunction of spleen-yang and accumulation of phlegm-dampness in the interior. Also indicated for cases of acute gastroenteritis, irritable colon, urinary infection and urinary calculi attributive to damage of vital energy by the combined attack of dampness and heat; for cases of edema due to chronic nephritis and ascites due to cirrhosis of liver, which are attributive to accumulation of dampness in the interior with formation of heat.

INTERPRETATION

The prescription is composed by the combination of Powder of Five Drugs Containing Poria (use Cortex Cinnamomi instead of Ramulus Cinnamomi) and Six to One Powder, and adding with Citri Grandis, Aucklandiae, Arecae and Zingiberis Recens. The Powder of Five Drugs Containing Poria has the effects of producing vital energy and promoting diuresis. The purpose of using Cortex Cinnamomi is to enhance the effect of warming urinary bladder. It is also applied for keeping the heart-fire and kidney-water in balance, warming yang and promoting diuresis when it is used together with Talcum. Six to One Powder has the effects of eliminating dampness-heat and discharging dampness by urination to relieve diarrhea. Since vital energy is essential for the fluid metabolism, Citri Grandis, Aucklandiae, Arecae and Zingiberis Recens are applied to promote the circulation of vital energy.

Decoction of Citri Grandis
and Bambusae in Taeniam
(Ju pi zhu ru tang)

INGREDIENTS

Exocarpium Citri Grandis	12g
Caulis Bambusae in Taeniam	15g
Radix Codonopsis Pilosulae	10g
Rhizoma Zingiberis Recens	10g
Radix Glycyrrhizae	3g
Fructus Ziziphi Jujubae	3 Pcs

All the above drugs are decocted in water for oral administration.

ACTION

Clearing away stomach-heat, stopping vomiting, strengthening spleen and regulating stomach; mainly for cases attributive to hypofunction of stomach and stomach-heat with adverse rising of gas, manifested as hiccup or vomiting, tender and red tongue, rapid and feeble pulse.

INDICATIONS

1. Also indicated for cases of morning sickness attributive to hypofunction of stomach complicated by stomach-heat.

2. By adding Poria, Rhizoma Pinelliae, Radix Ophiopogonis and folium Eriobotryae to this prescription, Decoction of Citri Grandis and Bambusae in Taeniam for Saving Lives is formed. It has the effects of nourishing the stomach and stopping vomiting, and is indicated for cases with deficiency of stomach-yin and dysfunction of stomach which are manifested as vomiting or hiccup, thirst, anorexia, tender and red tongue with a small amount of dry fur, small and rapid pulse, etc. As compared with the original prescription, it is better for nourishing the stomach and suitable for cases with vomiting caused by deficiency of stmach-yin and severe asthenia-heat.

3. By adding Calyx Kaki and omitting Codonopsis Pilosulae, Glycyrrhizae, Ziziphi Jujubae, another prescription named Newly Decoction of Citri Grandis and Bambusae in Taeniam is formed. It also has the effects of clearing away stomach-heat and stopping vomiting, but is indicated for cases of hiccup due to stomach-heat when the stomach-energy is not yet deficient.

4. Also applicable to cases of acute or chronic gastritis, duodenal ulcer and cholecystitis with vomiting, and protracted hiccup after abdominal operation which are attributive to hypofunction of stomach with stomach-heat and adverse rising of gas.

INTERPRETATION

Citri grandis regulates vital energy and stops vomiting; Bambusae in Taeniam clears away heat evil and stops vomiting. Two drugs used together may enhance the effects of bringing the adverse gas downward and stopping vomiting, and may clear away the stomach-heat without damaging the spleen-yang. Zingiberis Recens helps Bambusae in Taeniam to stop vomiting and cleat away stomach-heat, and inhibits its cold effect. Codonopsis Pilosulae has the effects of strengthening the spleen and regulating the stomach. Glycyrrhizae and Ziziphi Jujubae benefit vital energy and help Codonopsis Pilosulae to tonify middle-jiao energy, but their sweet taste interfere the anti-emetic effect and should be used in small dosage.

Decoction of Coptidis
(Huang lian tang)

INGREDIENTS

Rhizoma Coptidis	10g
Ramulus Cinnamomi	10g
Rhizoma Zingiberis	10g
Rhizoma Pinelliae (washed)	10g
Radix Codonopsis Pilosulae	6g
Radix Clycyrrhizae Praeparata	3g
Fructus Ziziphi Jujubae	6 Pcs

All the above drugs are decocted in water for oral administration.

ACTION

Regulating cold and heat, regulating the function of stomach and lowering down the adverss rising energy; mainly for cases attributive to heat in the chest and cold in the gastrointestine, which are manifested as feeling of heat and oppression over the chest, vomiting, abdominal pain, white and smooth fur on the tongue and wiry pulse.

INDICATIONS

1. Applicable to cases of watery diarrhea with increased gurgling sounds, abdominal pain, nausea, vomiting, vexation, thirst, yellow and greasy fur, soft and floating, smooth pulse, which are attributive to dampness-heat of intestines and stomach (predominantly dampness).

2. Indicated for cases characterized by a feeling of gas rushing up through the thorax to the throat from the lower abdomen, accompanied with irritability, dry mouth but without desire to drink, white and greasy fur on the tongue, wiry pulse, which are attributive to incoordination between the liver and the spleen, cold and heat, ascending and descending actions.

3. Also applicable to cases of duodenal ulcer, acute gastroenteritis, cholecystitis, or diarrhea attributive to heat in the upper and cold in the lower, or stagnation of dampness-heat in the intestines and stomach; or cases of hysteria and gastroenteric neurosis marked by feeling of gas rushing upward to the chest and thorax, which are attributive to incoordination between the liver and the

spleen.

INTERPRETATION

Copitis serves to clear away heat from the chest, and Zingiberis to expel cold from the gastrointestines. Their actions match with each other although their properties are entirely different. Pinelliae can ease the middle jiao when used together with Coptidis, and can regulate stomach and spleen and stop vomiting when used together with Zingiberis. Ramulus Cinnamomi serves to warm the middle jiao and expel cold when used together with Zingiberis and to regulate vital energy and lower down the adverse rising energy when used together with Pinelliae. Codonopsis Pilosulae, Glycyrrhizae Praeparata and Ziziphi Jujubae calm the middle jiao and regulate the function of spleen and stomach. In sum, the prescription aims at regulating cold and heat, especially at warming middle jiao and expelling cold.

Decoction of Evodia Fruit
(Wu zhu yu tang)

INGREDIENTS

Fructus Evodiae	3g
Radix Ginseng	6g
Fructus Zinziphi Jujubae	4 Pcs
Rhizoma Zingiberis Recens	18g

All the above drugs are decocted in water for administration.

INDICATIONS

Warming the middle-warmer and restoring qi, sending down the ascending reverse flow of qi to arrest vomiting.

Cold syndrome due to yang insufficiency of the liver and stomach manifested by the tendency to vomiting after meals, fullness and stuffiness in the chest; or by epigastralgia and gastric discomfort with acid regurgitation. Headache due to jueyin channel syndrome characterized by retching, salivation, and pain and cold feeling in the vertex. Vomiting and diarrhea due to shaoyin syndrome marked by symptoms such as cold extremities, dysphoria, etc.

The modified recipe can be applied to the treatment of such diseases as chronic gastritis, acute gastritis, gastroduodenal ulcer, hepatitis and others that pertain to cold syndrome due to yang insufficiency of the liver and stomach and with turbid yin reversing upwargs.

NOTE

1. The recipe should never be administered to patients with stomachache or vomiting of bitter fluid due to stagnated heat, as well as acid regurgitation that is ascribed to heat syndrome.

3. In a few patients, vomiting of the drug may become worse but it will subside by itself in half an hour. The patients should be advised to take a little rest after taking the drug to alleviate the reaction.

Decoction of Four Noble Drugs
(Si jun zi tang)

INGREDIENTS

Radix Ginseng	10g
Rhizoma Atractyiodis Macrocephalae	9g
Poria	9g
Radix Glycyrrhizae Praeparata	6g

All the ingredients are to be decocted in water for oral administration.

INDICATIONS

Replenishing qi and strengthening the spleen.

Qi-deficiency syndrome of the spleen and stomach with symptoms such as poor appetite, watery stool, pale complexion, low and weak voice, lassitude of limbs, thready weak or deep and loose pulse.

The recipe can be modified to treat deficiency of qi of the spleen and stomach as seen in cases of indigestion, chronic gastroenteritis, anemia, hypoproteinemia, chronic dysentery and various chronic disorders.

NOTE

1. Prolonged administration of the recipe may lead to symptoms of dry mouth and tongue, thirst, restlessness and so on.

2. The recipe should be administered with great care or not at all administered to those with high fever, or hyperactivity of fire due to yin deficiency, or

fullness due to stagnated qi, or insufficiency of body fluid, or excessive thirst and constipation.

INTERPRETATION

Of the four ingredients in the recipe, Ginseng possesses the effect of invigorating primordial qi and acts as a principal drug to strengthen the spleen and nourish the stomach. Bighead atractylodes rhizome is effective for strengthening the spleen and eliminating dampness and is considered as an assistant drug. Poria exerts the part of an adjuvant drug in achieving the effect of strengthening the spleen. Prepared licorice root is used as a guiding drug for regulating the middle-warmer.

Modern studies have confirmed that the recipe is effevtive for stimulating the central nervous system, facilitating the functional activities, promoting metabolism, digestion and absorption, regulating gastrointestinal functions, arresting diarrhea, and relieving swelling and inducing diureis.

Decoction of Gardeniae and Sojae Praeparatum
(Zhi zi chi tang)

INGREDIENTS

Fructus Gardeniae	10g
Semen sojae Praeparatum	12g

ACTION

Discharging the stagnated heat and relieving irritability; mainly for cases attributive to stagnation of heat in the chest, which manifest as fever, irritability, insomnia, feeling of oppression over the chest and epigastrium, red tongue with yellowish fur, rapid pulse.

INDICATIONS

1. For cases mentioned above accompanied with vomiting which is resulting from damage of the stomach by erroneous application of purgative or emetic, add Rhizoma Zingiberis Recens to regulate the stomach and stop vomiting. For those accompanied with feeling of fullness over the chest and abdomen resulting from damage of the spleen by erroneous application of purgative.

2. Applicable to cases of jaundice with bright yellow coloration of the skin,

fever, thirst, irritability, oliguria with yellow urine, of constipation, yellow and smooth fur on the tongue, wiry and rapid pulse, which are atributive to attack of dampness-heat (predominantly heat) to the liver and gallbladder.

3. Also applicable to cases of upper respiratory infection, esophagitis, vegetative nervous disorder and chronic gastritis with fever and irritability, which are attributive to the stagnation of heat in the chest; to cases of acute iterus infectious hepatitis and cholecystitis with jaundice attributive to the attack of dampness-heat; and to cases of chronic rhinitis, epidemic hemorrhagic fever, which are attributive to the stagnation of heat in the lung.

INTERPRETATION

Gardeniae is effective for clearing away heat and relieving irritability. Sojae Praeparatum, when used together with Gardeniae, is good for discharging the stagnated heat in the chest. Although its ingredients are small in number but it is effective for the purpose mentioned, and many prescriptions are developed from it in the later generations.

Decoction of Gentian for Purging Liver-fire
(Long dan xie gan tang)

INGREDIENTS

Radix Gentianae	6g
Radix Scutellariae	9g
Fructus Gardeniae	9g
Rhizoma Alismatis	12g
Caulis Akebiae	9g
Semen Plantaginis	9g
Radix Angelicae Sinensis	3g
Radix Rehmanniae	9g
Radix Bupleuri	6g
Radix Glycyrrhizae	6g

All the above drugs should be decocted in water for oral administration.

INDICATIONS

Purging excessive fire from the liver and gallbladder and removing damp-heat from the lower-warmer.

Upward attack of excessive fire in the liver and gallbladder or downward flow of damp-heat from the liver channel manifested as headache, conjunctival congestion, hypochondriac pain, bitter taste, deafness, pain and bulge of eat; or marked by stranguria with turbid urine, and damp-heat leukorrhagia.

Epually, the recipe can be modified to cure diseases marked by extreme fire in the liver and gallbladder, such as hypertension, vegetative nerve functional disturbance, acute conjunctivitis, acute otitis media, furuncle of nasal vestibule or furuncle of external auditory canal, acute cholecystitis and acute hepatitis; and to deal with cases with downward flow of damp-heat as seen in acute infection in the urinary system, acute orchitis, epididymitis, acute pelvic inflammation.

Since most of the drugs in the recipe are bitter in flavour and cold in property, constant and long-term administration of it is not advisable. Great care should be taken when exhibiting the drugs for those whose spleen-stomach functions are weak, otherwise the stomach-qi might be easily hurt.

INTERPRETATION

In the recipe, Gentian root extremely bitter in flavour and cold in nature, is used to purge excessive fire in the liver and gallbladder and clear damp-heat in the lower-warmer, providing the principal curative efficacy. Scutellaria root and capejasmine fruit being bitter in flavour and cold in nature, are used in combination to reinforce the effect of Gentian root playing the role of an assistant drug. Functioning together as adjuvant and guiding drugs. Oriental water plantain, fiveleaf akebia stem and plantain seed have the effect of removing heat and inducing diuresis to dispel damp-heat, while Chinese angelica root and dried rehmannia root possess the effect of nourishing yin and blood so as to soothe the liver. Bupeurun root and licorice root work in combination as guiding drugs, with the former having the effect of soothing the liver and regulating the circulation of qi in the liver and gallbladder and inducing the efficacy of all the medicines into the liver and gallbladder, and the latter having the effect of coordinating the effect of various ingredients in the recipe so as to prevent the stomach from being hurt by the bitter and cold property of the drugs.

Clinically and experimentally, it is ascertained that the recipe has the effect of bringing down the fever, tranquilizing the mind, relieving inflammation, inducing diuresis, resisting bacteria, promoting the function of gallbladder, protecting the liver, arresting bleeding and decreasing blood pressure.

Decoction of Glycyrrhizae and Zingiberis
(Gan cao gan jiang tang)

INGREDIENTS

Radix Glycyrrhizae Praeparata	12g
Rhizoma Zingiberis	10g

ACTION

Strengthening spleen-yang; mainly for cases attributive to deficiency of spleen-yang and stomach-yang, which manifest as chilliness, spontaneous sweating, cold limbs, flat taste in the mouth, no thirst, pale tongue with white and smooth fur, slow pulse.

INDICATIONS

1. For cases of hematemesis with pale complexion, profuse sweating over the head, cold breathing, cold limbs, slow pulse, which are attributive to the deficiency-cold of spleen and stomach and failure of keeping the blood inside the vessels, roasted Ginger is used instead of dried Ginger to enhance the effect of warming middle jiao and stopping bleeding.

2. Applicable to cases with abdominal pain which can be alleviated by warmth and aggravated by coldness, increased secretion of saliva, discharge of watery urine, white and smooth fur on the tongue, wiry and tense pulse, which are attributive to involvement of yang during exogenous febrile diseases.

3. Also indicated for consumptive pulmonary diseases manifested as cough with foamy expectoration, no thirst, dizziness, chilliness, pale tongue with white fur, slow pulse, which are attributive to the yang -deficiency of upper jiao and asthenia-cold of lung-energy.

4. Also applicable to cases of peptic ulcer, chronic gastritis, prolapse of gastric mucosa, etc. marked by cold limbs, sweating, or hematemesis, or abdominal pain, which are attributive to deficiency of spleen-yang and stomach-yang; and to cases of chronic obstructive emphysema and pulmonary abscess attributive to asthenia-cold of lung-energy.

INTERPRETATION

Glycyrrhizae has the effect of benefiting middle-jiao energy, and Zingiberis serves to warm the middle jiao and expel cold. The two drugs used together can strengthen spleen-yang to eliminate cold.

Decoction of Inula and Red Ochre
(Xuanfu Daizhe Tang)

INGREDIENTS

Flos Inulae (Wrapped with a piece of cloth when the decoction is being made)   9g

Ochra Haematitum	15g
Rhizoma Pinelliae	9g
Rhizoma Zingiberis Recens	9g
Radix Ginseng	6g
Fructus Ziziphi Jujubae	4 Pcs
Radix Glycyrrhizae Praeparata	6g

Decocted in water for oral administration.

INDICATIONS

Lowering the adverse flow of qi and resolving phlegm, invigorating qi and regulating the function of the stomach.

Syndrome of the deficient stomach-qi with reversed flow of qi marked by epigastric fullness and rigidity, frequent eructation, vomiting, salivation, white smooth fur of the tongue, taut and feeble pulse.

Chronic gastritis, gastroptosis, gastric dilatation, ulcerous pylorospasm or incomplete pylorochesis, neurogenic hiccup or vomiting, Meniere's disease and others marked by the symptoms of deficient stomach-qi with reversed flow of qi can be treated by the modified recipe.

INTERPRETATION

Inula flower in the recipe lowers the adverse flow of qi and expels phlegm, softens hard mass in the abdomen and relieves flatulence, and Red ochre functions in lowering the adverse flow of qi and promoting expectoration. The two drugs mentioned above act as principal drugs. Pinellia tuber and Fresh ginger as assistant drugs, expel phlegm, lower the adverse flow of qi, relieve flatulence and resolve mass. The last three drugs invigorate qi, regulate the function of stomach, coordinate the effects of all the other ingredients and act as adjuvant and guiding drugs.

Modern researches have proved that the recipe can produce the effects of tranquilizing the mind, relieving cough, expelling phlegm, arresting vomiting, relieving spasm of bronchial smooth muscle, protecting gastric mucosa and promoting the reproduction of the red blood cells and hemoglobin.

Decoction of Evodia Fruit
(Wu zhu yu tang)

INGREDIENTS

Fructus Evodiae	3g
Radix Ginseng	6g
Rhizoma Zingiberis Recens	18g
Fructus Ziziphi Jujubae	4pcs

INDICATIONS

Warming the middle-warmer and restoring qi, sending down the ascending reverse flow of qi to arrest vomiting. Cold syndrome due to yang insufficiency of the liver and stomach manifested by the tendency to vomiting after meals, fullness and stuffiness in the chest; or by epigastralgia and gastric discomfort with acid regurgitation. Headache due to jueyin channel syndrome characterized by retching, salivation, and pain and clod feeling in the vertex. Vomiting and diarrhea due to shaoyin syndrome marked by symptoms such as cold extremities , dysphoria, etc.

The modified recipe can be aplied to the treatment of such diseases as chronic gastritis, acute gastritis, gastrodue denal ulcer, hepatitis and others that pertain to clod syndrome due to yang insuffficiency of the liver and stomach and with turbid yin reversing upwards.

INTERPRETATION

In the recipe, Evodia fruit attributes to the channels of the spleen, liver and kidney. As a principal drugs, it is effective for the treatment of diseases in the three channels. It also has the functions of warming the stomach, sending down the reversed ascending qi to prevent vomiting, dispersing the depressed liver-energy to alleviate pain and warming the kidney to arrest diarrhaea. Ginseng is used as tonic for tonifying primordial qi and replenishing yin, and is considered as an assistant drug. Fresh ginger, with its pungent and warm property and its effect on the stomach, is administered as an adjuvant drug to lower the adverse flow of qi and reinforce the efficacy of the principal drug in arresting vomiting and scattering cold. Chinese-dates, as a guiding drug, has sweet flavor and slow effect and functions in the regulation of the middle-warmer. In not only relieves the dryness caused by the pungent and warm evodia fruit and fresh ginger, but also aids ginseng in festoring qi and strengthening the body's resistance.

Modern studies have showed that this recipe produces the effect of promoting blood circulation in the digestive tract, lowering tension of the smooth muscle, decreasing peristalsis, relieving spasm, preventing vomiting, alleviating pain, facilitating digestion, strengthening the functions of the whole body and so on.

Decoction of Magaoliae
officinalis and Other Two Drugs
(Hou po san wu tang)

INGREDIENTS

Cortex Magnoliae Officinalis	15g
Radix et Rhizoma Rhei (decocted later)	12g
Fructus Aurantii Immaturus	12g

ACTION

Activating vital energy, relieving abdominal fullness and inducing bowel movement; mainly for cases attributive to stagnation of vital energy and sluggishness of intestinal peristalsis, which manifest as abdominal flatulence, abdominal pain and tenderness, constipation, yellow and greasy fur on the tongue, sunken and wiry or sunken, unsmooth and strong pulse, etc.

INDICATIONS

Applicable to cases of dysentery with difficulty in defecation, abdominal pain and flatulence, yellow and greasy fur on the tongue, smooth pulse, which are attributive to the retention of dampness-heat.

Also applicable to cases of simple intestinal obstruction, cholecystitis, pancreatitis, etc. marked by abdominal fullness and constipation, which are attributive to stagnation of vital energy and sluggishness of intestinal peristalsis; and to cases of acute gastroenteritis, acute bacillary dysentery, marked by abdominal pain and diarrhea, which are attributive to retention of dampness-heat.

INTERPRETATION

Magnoliae Officinalis has the effects of relieving abdominal fullness and promoting bowel movement, and used in large dose as the chief drug. Rhei is decocted later and exerts a purgative action which is enhanced by Magnoliae Officinalis. Aurantii Immaturus is applied for expelling the stagnated energy. All the above three drugs used together serve to promote the circulation of vital energy and increase bowel movement, so as to relieve abdominal flatulence. The composition of this prescription is as same as the Decoction for Mild Purgation, but the dosage of the chief drugs are different. In the latter prescription, Rhei serves as the chief drug and is used in large dose, so that its action is chefly heat-eliminating and purgative; while in this prescription, a large dose of Magnoliae Officinalis is applied as the chief drug, and it chiefly serves to promote the circulation of vital energy and relieve abdominal flatulence.

Decoction of Magnoliae Officinalis
for Warming Middle Jiao
(Hou po wen zhong tang)

INGREDIENTS

Cortex Magnoliae Officinalis (prepared with ginger)	12g
Exocarpium citri Grandis	10g
Poria	10g
Rhizoma Zingiberis	6g
Semen Alpiniae	6g
Radix Aucklandiae	6g
Radix Glycyrrhizae Praeparata	3g
Rhizoma Zingiberis Recens	3 Pcs

All the above drugs should be decocted in water, for oral administration.

ACTION

Warming middle jiao, regulating vital energy, drying dampness and relieving fullness; mainly for abdominal flatulence due to cold-dampness of spleen and stomach and dysfunction of vital energy, or intermittent stomachache due to exogenous cold evil attacking the stomach.

INDICATIONS

1. The prescriprion is usually applied for cases of abdominal flatulence or pain dur to over taking of raw and cold foods and damage of middle jiao by cold evil, when both the healthy energy and the evil are hyperactive.

2. For cases of diarrhea with abdominal flatulence attributive to cold-dampness of spleen and stomach with stagnation of vital energy, subtract Glycyrrhizae and add Semen Arecae and Rhizoma Atractylodis to relieve flatulence and dry dampness.

3. For cases of leukorrhagia with thin discharge and fullness of the lower abdomen, which are attributive to downward attack of cold-dampness, subtract Zingiberis Recens and Glycyrrhizae Praeparata and add Rhizoma Atractylodis Macrocephalae and Ramulus Cinnamomi to warm middle jiao and eliminate dampness.

4. Also applicable to cases of gastritis, dyspepsia, peptic ulcer, intestinal tuberculosis, cervicitis, vaginitis, etc. marked by abdominal flatulence, or abdominal pain, or diarrhea, or leukorrhagia, which are attributive to cold-dampness of spleen and stomach.

INTERPRETATION

Magnosiaae Officinalis prepared with ginger is an important drug for relieving flatulence and applied in large dosage. it serves to warm middle jiao and lower the abnormal rising of energy. Zingiberis Recens, acrid in taste and hot in nature, enhances the action of Magnoliae Officinalis. Alpiniae, Citri Grandis, Aucklandiae are bitter in taste and warm in nature, and have the effects of drying dampness, promoting circulation of vital energy and easing middle jiao, so as to enhance the curative effects of Magnoliae Officinalis and Zingiberis. Poria can eliminate dampness and strengthen the spleen; Glycyrrhizae praeparata and Zingiberis Recens activate spleen-yang. All the above drugs used together can eliminate cold-dampness, promote the circulation of vital energy, and restore the function of spleen and stomach, leading to the subsidence of flatulence.

Decoction of Magnoliae Officinalis, Zingiberis Recens, Pinelliae, etc.
(Hou po sheng jiang ban xia gan cao ren shen tang)

INGREDIENTS

Magnoliae Officinalis Praeparata	10g
Rhizoma Zingiberis recens	10g
Rhizoma Pinelliae (washed)	10g
Radix Codonopsis Pilosulae	6g
Radix Glycyrrhizae Praeparata	5g

ACTION

Strengthening the spleen, benefiting the stomach, soothing the middle jiao and relieving fullness; mainly for cases attributive to hypofunction of spleen and stagnation of vital energy, which manifest as abdominal flatulence, poor appetite, tiredness, pale tongue with white and smooth fur, soft, floating and slow pulse.

INDICATIONS

1. Applicable to cases of diarrhea attributive to hypofunction of spleen and accumulation of dampness, which manifest as watery diarrhea, abdominal fullness, poor appetite, Sallow complexion, spiritlessness, fatigue, pale tongue with white and greasy fur, slow and weak pulse.

2. For cases atributive to hypofunction of spleen and abnormal rising of phlegm-dampness, which manifest as vomiting, pale complexion, fatigue, dizziness, palpitation, white and greasy fur, Smooth pulse. The dosage of Zingiberis Recens and Pinelliae may be increased to 12g, and those of Glycyrrhizae Praeparata and Codonopsis Pilosulae decreased to 3g.

3. Also applicable to cases of peptic ulcer, chronic cholecystitis, pancreatitis, gastritis, etc. marked by vomiting or abdominal fullness, which are attributive to hypofunction of spleen and stagnation of vital energy; and to cases of atrophic gastritis, pancreatic steatorrhea, chronic colitis, etc. marked by diarrhea,

which are attributive to hypofunciton of spleen and accumulation of dampness.

INTERPRETATION

Magnoliae Officinalis Praeparata and Pinelliae used together can promote the circulation of vital energy and lower the adverse rising energy, so as to relieve intestinal stagnation and abdominal flatulence. Codonopsis Pilosulae and Glycyrrhizae Praeparata are used for strengthening the spleen and stomach. Zingiberis Recens is used for activating the spleen-yang and decreasing the toxicity of Pinelliae.

Decoction of Pinellia and Magnolia Bark
(Ban xia hou po tang)

INGREDIENTS

Rhizoma Pinelliae	12g
Cortex Magnoliae Officinalis	9g
Poria	12g
Rhizoma Zingiberis Recens	9g
Folium Perillae	6g

Decocted in water for oral; administration.

INDICATIONS

Promoting the circulation of qi to alleviate mental depression, lowering the adverse flow of qi and resolving phlegm.

Globus hystericus marked by a subjective sensation as if a plum pit is stuck in the throat which can neither be thrown up nor swallowed down, or accompanied by fullness and distress in the chest and hypochondrium, or cough or vomiting, white, moist or greasy fur of the tongue, and slippery or taut pulse.

Pharyngoneurosis, pharyngitis, edema of plica vocalis, bronchitis, bronchial asthma, neurogenic vomiting, gastric neurosis and vomiting of pregnancy marked by stagnancy of phlegm and qi or reversed flow of qi can be treated by the modified recipe.

The recipe is mainly composed of drugs bitter and pungent in taste, warm and dry in nature, so it is only indicated for stagnation of phlegm and qi, partially for the phlegm-dampness. It is contraindicated in patients with deficiency of yin-fluid of hyperactivity of pathogenic fire due to yin deficiency.

INTERPRETATION

Pinellia tuber in the recipe, with a pungent flavor and warm nature, is used as a principal drug to resolve phlegm, disperse stagnancy and regulate the stomach and lower the adverse flow of qi. Magnolia brak, pungent in flavor, bitter in taste and warm in nature, can achieve the effects of sending down the ascending qi, relieving the sensation of fullness and assisting Pinellia tuber in dispersing stagnation and lowering the adverse flow of qi. Poria, sweet and bland in taste, can be used to induce diuresis and assist Pinellia tuber in resolving phlegm. The two drugs are regarded as assistant drugs. Fresh ginger, pungent in flavor and warm in nature, can be used to disperse stagnation, regulate the stomach and relieve vomiting. Perilla leaf promotes the circulation of qi, soothes the liver and regulates the spleen by means of its aroma. The two drugs are used as adjuvant drugs.

Modern researches have proved that the recipe has the effects of expelling phlegm, arresting cough, relieving spasm of smooth muscles of bronchus and regulating the function of autonomic nerve and removing edema.

Decoction of Pinelliae for Purging Stomach-Fire
(Ban xia xie xin tang)

INGREDIENTS

Rhizoma Pinelliae Praeparata	12g
Rhizoma Zingiberis	10g
Radix Scutellariae	10g
Radix Codonopsis Pilosulae	10g
Rhizoma Coptidis	6g
Radix Glycyrrhizae Praeparata	6g
Fructus Ziziphi Jujubae	6 Pcs

ACTION

Dispersing cold-dampness, purging heat strengthening the spleen and regulating the stomach; mainly for cases attributive to the attack of dampness-heat to the gastrointestines, manifested as abdominal fullness without pain, vomiting or retching, increased gurgling sound, diarrhea, thin and yellow, greasy fur on the tongue, wiry and rapid pulse.

INDICATION

1. For cases of diarrhea with yellow, thick and greasy fur on the tongue, attributive to severe dampness-heat, add Radix Puerariae and Semen Arecae and omit Codonopsis Pilosulae and glycyrrhizae; for cases with frequent vomiting, also omit codonopsis Pilosulae and Glycyrrhizae and use Rhizoma Zingiberis Recens instead of Zingiberis.

2. Also applicable to cases of chronic gastroenteritis, peptic ulcer, infantile dyspepsia with vomiting and diarrhea, which are attributive to the stagnation of dampness and heat evil with dysfunction of stomach-energy.

INTERPRETATION

Pinelliae acts with Zingiberis to warm and disperse the cold-dampness evil; Scutellariae and Coptidis purge the heat from the interior. All the above four drugs serve as the principal drugs in the prescription. Codonopsis Pilosulae, Ziziphi Jujubae and Glycyrrhizae have the effects of strengthening the spleen and stomach and restoring their function of absorption and digestion. As a whole, the prescription applies both bitter and acrid drugs to eliminate dampness and heat evil, both cold and hot drug to regulate yin and yang, both tonifying and purging drugs to deal with asthenia and sthenia syndrome.

Decoction of Puerariae for Alcoholism
(Ge hua jie cheng tang)

INGREDIENTS

Radix Aucklandiae	1. 5g
Radix Codonopsis Pilosulae	6g
Polyporus Umbellatus	6g
Poria	6g
Exocarpium Citri Grandis	6g
Semen Amoni	6g
Rhizoma Atractylodis Macrocephalae	10g
Rhizoma Zingiberis	10g

Massa Fermentata Medicinalis(fried)	10g
Rhizoma Alismatis	10g
Pericarpium Citri Reticulatae	10g
Fructus Amomi Cardamomi	10g
Flos Puerariae	12g

INDICATIONS

Eliminating alcoholic dampness, and strengthening the spleen and stomach; mainly for cases of alcoholism manifested as dizziness, vomiting, feeling of oppression over the chest, anorexia, fatigue, oliguria, hoose stools, pale tongue with white and smooth fur, slow pulse, which are attributive to damage of the spleen and stomach by alcoholic dampness.

Applicable to cases of acute alcoholism, indigestion, chronic cholecystitis, duodenal ulcer, chronic pancreatitis, cirrhosis of liver (caused by alcoholism), malnutritional edema, etc. which are attributive to hypofunction of spleen with retention of dampness.

INTERPRETATION

Flos Puerariae can relieve alcoholism and eliminate alcoholic dampness from the superficies; Poria, Polyporus Umbellatus and Alismatis promote diuresis, and eliminate dampness from the urine. They keep each other to accomplish the elimination of alcoholic dampness from the body. Amomi, Aucklandiae, Amomi Cardamomi, Citri Reticulatae and Citri Grandis are applied to regulate vital energy, soothe the middle jiao and eliminate dampness. Among them, Amomi can also treat alcoholism when it is used together with Massa Fermentata Medicinalis, and enhances the anti-alcoholic effect of Flos Puerariae. Codonopsis Pilosulae, Zingiberis and Atractylodis Macrocephalae can warm middle jiao and strengthening the spleen.

<h1>Decoction of Puerariae,
Scutellariae and coptidis
(Ge gen huang qin huang lian tang)</h1>

INGREDIENTS

Radix Puerariae	20g
Radix Scutellariae	10g
Rhizoma Coptidis	10g
Radix Glycyrrhizae Praeparate	3g

ACTION

Clearing away interior heat evil and expelling the superficial evils from the body sufrace; mainly for cases with exogenous superficial evil not yet eliminated but the heat evil already attacking the interior, which are manifested as fever, diarrhea with foul discharge, burning sensation over the anus, thirst, yelllow for on the tongue and rapid pulse.

INDICATIONS

This prescription is chiefly for clearing away the interior heat and also for e-liminating superficial evils from the body surface, and is suitable for diarrhea or dysentery no matter the superficies-syndrome is present or not.

Also applicable to cases with fever and diarrhea occurring in common cold of gastrointestinal type, acute enteritis, fulminant dyspepsia, typhoid, etc., which are attributive to heat in both superficies and interior; also for cases of stomatitis and periodontitis, attributive to stomach-heat.

INTERPRETATION

Puerariae has the effects of expelling the superficial evil to lower the fever and of rising the spleen and stomach energy and dctivating lucid yang to arrest diarrhea; Coptis and Scutellariae which are bitter and cold have the effects of ex-pelling the heat and dampness evil of spleen and stomach; glycyrrhiza praeparata with sweet test and mild nature has the effects of regulating middle jiao and pre-venting Scutellaria and Coptidis from damaging the stomach. All the above drugs used together serve to expel the evil factors from both the superficies and the in-terior.

Decoction of Rhubarb and Aconite
（Da huang fu zi tang）

INGREDIENTS

Radix et Rhizoma Rhei	9g
Radix Aconiti Praeparata	9g
Herba Asari	3g

Decocted in water for oral administration. Generally, the dosage of rhubarb should not exceed that of prepared aconite root.

INDICATIONS

Warming yang and dispelling pathogenic cold, relieving constipation and promoting the circulation of qi.

Syndrome of interior excess due to the accumulation of pathogenic cold, manifested as abdominal pain, constipation, hypochondriac pain, fever, cold limbs, white and greasy coating on the tongue, taut and tense pulse. Besides, this recipe can be modified to deal with such cases as acute or chronic constipation accompanied with accumulation of pathogenic cold, acute appendicitis, intestinal obstruction ascribable to insufficient-cold type.

If the administration of this recipe results in the relief of constipation, the patient can be pronounced to be out of danger; but if the patient does not respond well to the recipe marked by constipation, vomiting, cold limbs and thready pulse, it indicates that patient is still in danger.

INTERPRETATION

Of the three ingredients in the recipe, Rhubarb and Prepared aconite root are both referred to as principal drugs, the first of which, acrid in flavour and extremely hot in nuture, has the functions of warming and recuperating the kidney-yang in order to remove constipation due to excessive cold as well as to relieve pain, while the second is used to remove pathogenic accumulation by purging the bowels. Asarum herb of acrid flavour and warm property is used as an assistant drug for expelling pathogenic cold from the channels and assisting in the functions of warming the kidney-yang and relieving pain. The cooperation of three drugs results in a warm nature with well preserved effects of removing retention and expelling accumulation of pathogen. So it is considered the very recipe for purging cold accumulation with drugs of warm nature.

Modern researches have proved that this recipe possesses the efficacies of promoting metabolism and blood circulation as well as cardiac stimulant, analgesia and purgation.

Decoction of Smaller Dosage of Pinelliae
(Xiao ban xia tang)

INGREDIENT

Rhizoma Pinelliae Praeparata	15g
Rhizoma Zingiberis Recens	12g

ACTION

Eliminating phlegm and stopping vomiting; mainly for cases of vomiting due to retention of phlegm in the stomach and adverse rising of turbid yin, which are accompanied with profuse expectoration, feeling of oppression over the chest, no thirst, smooth and greasy fur on the tongue.

INDICATIONS

1. For cases of morning sickness with whitish and smooth tongue fur, which are attributive to abnormal rising of phlegm-dampness.

2. For cases of chronic gastritis, gastric ulcer, hysteria, Meniere's syndrome, gastrointestinal neurosis, etc. marked by vomiting, which are attributive to retention of phlegm in the stomach and odverse rising of turbid yin.

INTERPRETATION

Pinelliae is the chief drug in this prescription, which has the effects of drying dampness, eliminating phlegm, lowering the abnormally rising energy and stopping vomiting. Zingiberis Recens serves to warm the spleen and kidney and expel dampness, lower the upward rising of turbid-yin and stop vomiting, and also inhibit the toxicity of Pinelliae.

Decoction of Three Kinds of Kernel
(San ren tang)

INGREDIENTS

Semen Armeniacae Amarum	15g
Talcum	18g
Tetrapanacis	6g
Semen Amoni Cardamoni	6g
Herba Lophatheri	6g
Cortex Magnoliae Officinalis	6g
Semen Coicis	18g
Rhizoma Pinelliae	10g

INDICATIONS

Promoting the functional activities of qi and eliminating dampness and heat.

Initial stage of infectious febrile disease due to dampness and heat marked by headache, chills, pain and heavy sensation of the body, slight yellow complexion, fullness in the chest and anorexia, afternoon fever, white fur, absence of thirst, and taut, thready and feeble pulse.

Acute gastroenteritis, acute hepatitis, influenza, pyelitis, typhoid fever and other cases related to the above syndrome with more dampness than heat can be treated by the modified recipe.

The recipe is contraindicated in patients with deficiency of yin-fluid, or fever due to yin deficiency. Damp-heat diseases with more manifestations of heat than dampness should be treated with great care.

INTERPRETATION

Bitter apricot kernel facilitates the flow of lung-qi in the upper-warmer. Round cardamon seed, as an aromatic, dispels dampness and promotes the circulation of qi to remove the stagnation in the middle-warmer. Coix seed sweet in taste and cold in nature, excretes dampness and heat to strengthen the spleen. Talc, Rice-paper pith and Lophatherum strengthen the effects of excreting dampness and clearing heat. Pinellia tuber and Magnolia bark can promote the circulation of qi to dispel dampness and relieve feeling of fullness in the upper adbdomen.

Modern researches have proved that the recipe is effective in strengthening the actions of allaying fever, regulating the function of the stomach and intestine, arresting vomiting and diarrhea, inducing diuresis, relieving inflammation and resisting bacteria.

Decoction of Yellow Dragon with Supplements
(Xin jia huang long tang)

INGREDIENTS

Radix Rehmanniae	15g
Radix Glycyrrhizae	6g
Radix Ginseng	4.5g
Radix et Rhizoma Rhei	9g
Natrii Sulphas	9g
Radix Scrophulariae	15g
Radix Ophiopogonis	15g
Radix Angelicae Sinensis	4.5g
Sea Cucumber	2 pieces
Ginger juice	6 spoonfuls

The above drugs should be decocted in water for oral administration. Ginseng should be decocted alone, and then poured into the decoction of other ingredients before intake.

INDICATIONS

Nourishing yin, replenishing the vital qi and purging the accumulation of pathogenic heat.

Syndrome of the accumulation of heat accompanied by weakened body resistance with such symptoms as constipation, abdominal fullness and distension, mental fatigue, shortness of breath, dryness of the mouth and throat, parched or chapped lips with fissures on the tongue, dry scorched yellow or black tongue fur.

Equally, this recipe can be modified to treat paralytic, simple and obliterative intestinal obstruction, habitual constipation, epidemic or non-epidemic febrile diseases in their climax marked by interior excess and accumulation of heat, and effective for those with deficiency of the vital qi and massive loss of yin and blood.

INTERPRETATION

In the recipe, Rhubarb and Mirabilite purge the bowels to remove heat, soften hardness and moisten dryness. Slim dried rehmannia root, scrophularia root, Ophiopgon root and sea cucumber nourish yin to increase the body fluid. Liquorice, ginseng and Chinese angelica root not only replenish the vital qi but also tonify yin and blood . As a result, the bowels are purged and pathogenic heat is expelled. Ginger juice can be used to nourish the stomach and spleen to send down the stomach-qi and prevent retch and vomiting.

Modern researches have confirmed that this recipe has the efficacies of relieving inflammation, resisting bacteria, improving intestinal blood circulation and intestinal peristalsis, increasing the activity of gastrointestinal tract, loosing the bowels, tranquilizing the mind and bringing eown fever.

Digestion Pill of Betel Nut
(Bing lang si xiao wan)

INGREDIENTS
Semen Arecae
Radix et Rhizoma Rhei
Semen Pharbitidis
Fructus Gleditsiae Abnormalis
Rhizoma Cyperi
Faeces Trogopterorum
Water-paste pills, 3g every 50 pills, 9g per packet.

ACTIONS
Promoting digestion to remove stagnated food, promoting circulation of qi to remove water retention by purgation.

INDICATIONS
Dyspepsia, phlegm retention, abdominal distention, eructation, acid regurgitation, constipation, etc.

DIRECTION

To be taken orally, 100 pills each time, twice a day.

Never administered to pregnant women or patients with loose stool due to insufficiency of the spleen.

Digestion-Promoting Pill
(Kai xiong shun qi wan)

INGREDIENTS

    Semen Arecae

    Semen Pharbitidis

    Pericarpium Citri Reticulatae

    Radix Aucklandiae

    Rhizoma Sparganii

    Rhizoma Zedoariae

    Fructus Gleditsiae Abnormalis

    Cortex Magnoliae Officinalis

Water-paste pills, 1g every 16 pills, 18g per packet

ACTIONS

Promoting digestion and removing stagnated food.

INDICATIONS

Indigestion, stagnation of qi, stuffiness in the chest, abdominal distention, epigastralgia, etc.

DIRECTION

To be taken orally, 3-9g each time, once or twice a day. No administration to pregnant women and careful administration to old and debilitated patients.

Ease Powder
(Xiao yao san)

INGREDIENTS

Radix Bupleuri	15g
Radix Angelicae Sinensis	15g
Radix Paeoniae Alba	15g

Poria	15g
Rhizoma Atractylodis Macrocephalae	15g
Rhizoma Zingiberis Recens Praeparata	a little
Herba Menthae	a little
Radix Glycyrrhizae Praeparate	6g

Grind the above drugs except Roasted ginger and peppermint into powder, take 6 to 9 grams each time with a decoction in small amount of roasted ginger and peppermint. If used as decoction the dosage can be reduced proportionally according to the orginal recipe.

INDICATIONS

Soothing the liver to disperse the depressed qi, and invigorating the spleen to nourish the blood.

Stagnation of the liver-qi with deficiency of the blood marked by hypochondriac pain, headache, dizziness, bitter mouth, dry throat, mental weatiness and poor appetite, or alternate attacks of chills and fever, or irregular menstruation, distension in the breast, light redness of the tongue, taut and feeble pulse.

Patients with chronic hepatitis, pleuritis, chronic gastritis, neurosis, irregular menstruation marked by the symptoms of stagnation of the liver-qi with deficiency of the blood can be treated by the modified recipe.

INTERPRETATION

Bupleurum root in the recipe soothes the liver to disperse the depressed qi. Chinese angelica root and white peony root nourish the blood and the liver. The joint use of the three drugs is able to treat the primary cause of stagnation of the liver-qi and deficiency of the blood. Poria and bighead atractylodes rhizome strengthen the middle-warmer and reinforce the spleen so as to enrich the source of growth and development of the qi and blood. Roasted ginger regulates the stomach and warms the middle-warmer. Peppermint assists bupleurum root in soothing the liver to disperse the depressed qi. Prepared licorice root can not only assist bighead atractylodes rhizome and Poria in replenishing qi and invigorating the middle-warmer but also coordinate the effects of all the drugs in the recipe.

Modern researches have proved that the recipe has the remarkable effects of nourishing the liver, tranquilzing the mind and relieving spasm. It is also effective in promoting digestion, coordinating uterine function, nourishing blood, strengthening the stomach.

Gastralgia Tablet (1)
(An wei pian)

INGREDIENTS

 Rhizoma Corydalis

 Alumen Exsiccatum

 Os sepiella seu Sepiae

Tablets, 0.4g each tablet, 100 tablets per bottle.

ACTIONS

Relieving gstric hyperacidity and alleviating stomachache.

INDICATIONS

Gastric or duodenal ulcer and chronic gastritis.

DIRECTION

To be taken orally, 5-7 tablets each time, 3-4 times a day

Gastralgia Tablet (2)
(Wei te ling pian)

INGREDIENTS

 Rhizoma Corydalis

 Alumen

Tablets, 0.35g each tablet (base).

ACTIONS

Relieving hyperacidity and gastralgia.

INDICATIONS

Gastric and duodenal ulcer, chronic gastritis.

DIRECTION

To be taken orally, 4-6 tablets each time, 3 times a day.

Gypsum Decoction
(Yu nu jian)

INGREDIENTS

Gypsum Fibrosum	30g
Rasic Rehmanniae Praeparata	30g
Radix Ophiopogonis	6g
Rhizoma Anemarrhenae	4.5g
Radix Achyranthis Bidentatae	4.5g

Decocted in water for oral administration, either warm or cold.

INDICATION

Clearing stomach-heat and nourishing yin.

Syndromes of stomach-heat and yin deficiency characterized by headache, toothache, odontoseisis, dysphoria with thirst, dry and reddened tongue with dry yellow coating.

The recipe can be modified for treating periodontitis, purulent swelling of gums, acute stomatitis, glossitis, chronic gastritis, indicating wyndromes of stomach-heat and yin deficiency.

INTERPRETATION

In the recipe, Gypsum, pungent and sweet in taste and extreme cold in nature, is used as a principal drug providing the effect of clearing stagnation of heat. Prepared rehmannia root, which is sweet and warm, acts as an assistant drug, giving the effect of invigoration yin. When Gypsum and Prepared rehmannia root are exhibited in combination, the effect of clearing pathogenic fire and nourishing the body fluid can be yielded, Wind-weed rhizome, bitter in taste and cold and moist in property, is used to reinforce the effect of Gypsum in purging pathogenic fire and heat from the stomach, and Ophiopogon root has the eftect of nourishing the stomach-yin and can aid Prepared rehmannia root in nourishing the kidney-yin. Achyranthes root functions in guiding pathogenic heat downwards to reduce eccessive fire .

Modern studies have revealed that this recipe possesses the efficacies of relieving inflammation, allaying fever, tranquilizing the mind, nourishing the body and consolidatiing the constitution.

Hemp Seed Pill
(Ma zi ren wan)

INGREDIENTS

Fructus Cannabis	500g
Radix Paeoniae Alba	250g
Fuctus Aurantii Immaturus	250g
Radix et Rhizoma Rhei	500g
Cortex Magnoliae Officinalis	250g
Semen Armeniacae Amarum	250g

The above drugs are ground into fine powder and then boluses are made out. Nine grams is taken each time orally with warm boiled water, one or two times a day.

INDICATIONS

Moistening the intestines to relieve constipation.

Syndrome of constipation due to intestinal dryness, manifested as frequency of urination, dry stool, or constipation due to dehydration after febrile diseases, and habitual constipation.

This recipe can equally be adapted for the treatment of constipation caused by intestinal dryness due to over-sweating in the febrile diseases, habitual constipation marked by rabbit-stool-like feces.

The recipe should be administered with great care for the aged and the weak or those with constipation caused by exhaustion of body fluid and blood dryness without pathogenic heat. It is not advisable for the pregnant women.

INTERPRETATION

This recipe, in fact, is the modified copy of Minor Decoction for Purging Down Digestive Qi, with its dosage reduced and with the addition of hemp seed, bitter apricot kernel, white peony root and honey. In the recipe, hemp seed great in dosage, sweet in flavour, mild in nature and abundant in lipid, functions as the principal drug, moisten the large intestine for treatment of constipation. The acrid and mild natured bitter apricot kernel, as an assistant drug, has the function of sending down qi and relaxing the bowels with its lubricant nature. All the ingredients in the Minor Decoction for Purging Down Digestive Qi have the effect of purging the retention of gastrointestinal dryness and heat, and thus being referred to as adjuvant drugs. The guiding drug is honey with effect of moistening dryness and relaxing the bowels. The various ingredients of the prescription act in coorperation to moisten the intestine and loose the bowels, and pertain to the recipe of mild laxation by moistening.

Modern researches have confirmed that this recipe has the functions of moistening the intestine and softening stool.

Lenitive Pill
(Bao he wan)

INGREDIENTS

Fructus Crataegi	180g
Massa Fermentata Medicinalis	60g
Rhizoma Pinelliae	90g
Poria	90g
Pericarpium Citri Reticulatae	30g
Fructus Forsythiae	30g
Semen Raphani	30g

The pills are prepared by grinding all the above drugs into very fine powder first and then refining powdered drugs with water, to be taken 6-9g each time with warm boiled water.

INDICATIONS

Promoting digestion and regulating the stomach. Retention of food due to improper diet with symptoms such as stuffiness and fullness in the epigastrium, distention in the abdomen with pain at times, acid regurgitation and eructation with fetid odor, loss of appetite, nausea, vomiting, or diarrhea, intermittent fever or dysentery dur to retention of food, greasy and yellowish coating of the tongue, and slippery pulse.

Equally, the above syndrome occurring in cases such as indigestion and gastroenteritis and others may be treated with the modified recipe.

The recipe should be administered with great care to patients with the insufficiency of spleen. Greasy and spicy food is prohibited during adminstration.

INTERPRETATION

In the recipe, hawthorn fruit considered as the principal drug, can be used to remove all kinds of food stagnancy. It is especially good at removing the stagnancy of greasy food. The second and the last drugs act in combination as assistant drugs, with former being effective for promoting digestion and strengthening the spleen, especially for removing stagnated food related to immoderate drinking, while the latter being contributive to keeping the adverse qi downward and promoting digestion, especially to removing the stagnated grain food. The rest act together as adjuvant drugs, of which Pinellia tuber and tangerine peel have the effect of promoting the flow of stomach-qi and removing the stagnated food, regulating the functions of stomach to arrest vomiting; Poria has the effects of strengthening the spleen and inducing diuresis, regulating the stomach and spleen to arrest diarrhea; and forsythia fruit has the effects of clearing away heat and scattering stagnacancy.

Modern studies have proved that this recipe possesses the efficacies for promoting digestion and peristalsis of the stomach and intestines, arresting vomiting, subduing inflammation and resisting bacteria.

Liver-benefiting Tablet
(Li gan pain)

INGREDIENTS
　　Bilis Porci
　　Herba Lysimachiae
Tablets, 0. 2g each one, 100 tablets per bottle.

ACTIONS
Removing heat and dampness from the liver and gallbladder.

INDICATIONS
Acute or chronic infectious hepatitis and cholecystitis, manifested as hypochondriac pain, jaundice, bitter sensation in the mouth, yellow urine, abdominal distention and loose stool.

DIRECTION
To be taken orally, 2-4 tablets each time, 3 times a day.

Liver-protecting Tablet
(Hu gan pian)

ENGREDIENTS

    Extractum Fructus Schisandrae

    Extractum Protectionis pro Hepate

    Herba Artemisiae Capillaris

    Radix Bupleuri

    Radix Isatidis

    Pulvis Bilis

Tablets, 0. 35g each tablet, 100 tablets per bottle; borehole packs in aluminium-foil: 12 tablets per strip, 4 strips each pack.

ACTIONS

Soothing the liver, regulating the circulation of qi, clearing away heat and dampness.

INDICATIONS

Stagnation of the liver-qi, manifested as distending pain in the hypochondrium, belching, poor appetite and others. It is used to treat chronic hepatitis, persisting hepatitis, cirrhosis and other troulbes in the liver. It is more effective in lowering transaminase.

DITECTION

To be taken orally, 4-6 tablets each time, 3 times a day for adults.

Contraindicated for patients with jaundice of yin type.

Liver-restoring Tablet
(Li gan long pian)

INGREDIENTS

    Radix Isatidis

    Radix Curcumae

    Herba Artemisiae Capillaris

    Fructus Schisandrae

    Radix Angelicae Sinensis

Radix Glycyrrhizae

Radix Astragali Seu Hedysari

Extractum Radicis Acanthopanacis Senticosi

Tablets, 0.3g each tablet, 60 tablets per bottle.

ACTIONS

Relieving the depressed liver, clearing away heat and removing dampness by diuresis, strengthening body resistance and restoring the normal functions of body.

INDICATIONS

Symptoms such as distending pain in hypochondrium, eructation and poor appetite caused by stagnation of the liver-qi. And clinically, acute hepatitis, hepatitis of persisting type, chronic active hepatitis. It markedly reduces G P T and I I and is effective for the conversion of HBsAg into negartiveness.

DIRECTION

To be taken orally with warm boiled water. For adults: 5 tablets each time, 3 times a day; for children, the doses should be reduced accordingly.

Liver-soothing Bolus
(Shu gan wan)

INGREDIENTS

Fructus Meliae Toosendan

Rhizoma Corydalis

Radix Paeoniae Alba

Rhizoma Curcumae Longae

Radix Aucklandiae

Lignum Aguilariae Resinatum

Fructus Amomi Rotundus

Fructus Amomi

Cortex Magnoliae Officinalis

Pericarpium Citri Reticulatae

Fructus Aurantii

Poria

Honeyed-boluses, 6g each bolus.

ACTIONS

Regulating the liver, normalizing the function of the stomach and regulating the flow of qi to alleviate pain.

INDICATIONS

Stagnation of the liver-qi, manifested as distention and fullness in the hypochondria, poor appetite, dyspepsia, epigastralgia, epigastric upset, vomiting, belching and pantothen. Also advisable for hepatitis, gastritis, gastro-duodenal ulcer and hysteria due to stagnation of the liver-qi.

DIRECTION

To be taken orally, 1 bolus each time, 2-3 times a day. It should be used with great care for patients in pregnancy.

Liver-soothing Infusion
(Shu gan chong ji)

INGREDIENTS

      Spica Prunellae

      Herba Atemisiae Capillaris

      Rhizoma Polygoni Cuspidati

      Radix Glycyrrhizae

      Baphicacanthus Cusia

      Herba Taraxaci

      Radix Bupleuri

      Rhizoma Imperatae

Medicinal granules (infusion), 20g each packet, 10 packets per box.

ACTIONS

Soothing the liver and regulating the circulation of qi, clearing away heat and toxic materials.

INDICATIONS

Acute icterohepatitis or non-icterohepatitis, also certain effective for chronic or persisting hepatitis.

DIRECTION

To be taken orally after being infused in boiling water, 1 packet each time, 3 times a day.

Liver-tonic Tablet
(Gan xi le)

INGREDIENTS

 Acidum Oleanolicum

 Extractum Fructus Schisandrae

 Extractum Radicis Acanthopanacis Senticosi

ACTIONS

Relieving the depressed liver and removing toxic substances, strengthening the body resistance and restoring the normal functioning of body to consolidate the constitution

INDICATIONS

Distension and pain in the hypochondrium, bitter taste, dry throat, poor appitite, loose stool, lassitude and weakness, restlessness and insomnia, soreness in the loins and knees. Various types of viral hepatitis such as acute icterohepatitis, chronic and active hepatitis, chronic persisting hepatitis, etc. Its has correcting function for positive signs of HBsAg.

DIRECTION

To be taken orally, 4 tablets or capsules each time, 3 times a day.

Tablets: Each tablet containing 10mg of oleanolic acid, 100 tablets per bottle.

Capsules: Each capsule containing 10mg of oleanolic acid, 60 capsules per bottle, 80 bottles per box.

Major Decoction of Bupleurum
(Da chai hu tang)

INGREDIENTS

Radix Bupleuri	15g
Radix Scutellariae	9g
Radix Paeoniae Alba	9g
Rhizoma Pinelliae	9g
Fructus Aurantii Immaturus Praeparata	9g
Radix et Rhizoma rhei	6g
Rhizoma Zingiberis Recens	15g
Fructus Ziziphi Jujubae	

All the drugs listed above are to be decocted in water twice, and after the residue is removed, the decoction is to be taken warm in two separate doses.

ACTION

Treating shaoyang disease by mediation and purging away internal stasis of heat.

INDICATIONS

Shaoyang and yangming diseases complex marked by alternate attacks of chills and fever, fullness and oppression in the chest, hypochondriac discomfort, frequent vomiting, mental depression and dysphoria, epigastric fullness and pain or epigastric rigidity, constipation or diarrhea due to interior cold and exterior heat, yellow tongue fur, stringy and forceful pulse.

Patients with acute cholecystitis, cholelithiasis, acute pancreatitis and infection of abdominal activity marked by the above-mentioned symptoms can be treated by the modified recipe.

Major Decoction for Purging Down Digestive Qi
(Da chen qi tang)

INGREDIENTS

Radix et Rhizoma Rhei (decocted later)	12g
Cortex Magnoliae Officinalis (decocted prior)	15g

Fructus Aurantii Immaturus (decocted prior)   12g

Natrli Sulfas (infused in)   9g

INDICATIONS

Expelling pathogenic heat and loosening the bowels, promoting the circulation of qi to purge accumulation in the bowels.

1. Excessive-heat syndrome of yangming-fu organ, manifested as constipation, frequent wind through the anus, feeling of fullness in the abdomen, abdominal pain with tenderness and guarding, tidal fever, delirium, polyhidrosis of hands and feet, prickled tongue with yellow dry fur or dry black tongue coating with fissures deep and forceful pulse.

2. Syndrome of fecal impaction due to heat with watery discharge, manifested as watery discharge of terribly foul odor accompanied by abdominal distension and pain with tenderness and guarding, dry mouth and tongue, smooth and forceful pulse.

3. Cold limbs due to excess of heat, convulsion, mania and other symptoms belonging to excess syndrome of interior heat.

Equally, this recipe can be modified to deal with infectious or non-infectious febrile diseases in their climax marked by accumulation of heat type, and in the treatment of paralytic, simple and obliterative intestinal obstructions.

INTERPRETATION

Rhei has the purgative effect and eliminating heat, but cannot induce an immediate purgation since it only promotes the peristalsis of large intestine and connot soften the dry feces. While Natrii Sulfas can creat a hypertonic condition in the large intestine and retain enough amount of water to soften the dry feces. Hence the two drugs used together may give an immediate purgation. Morever, Magnoliae Officinalis and Aurantii Immaturus have the effects of promoting vital energy circulation and relieving distension in the abdomen, so as to regulate the function of the gastrointestine, and enhance the effect of Rhei and Natrii Sulfas.

Minor Decoction for Purging Down Digestive Qi
(Xiao cheng qi tang)

INGREDIENTS

Radix et Rhizoma Rhei (decocted later)	12g
Cortex Magnoliae Offficinalis	6g
Fructus Aurantii Immaturus	9g

INDICATIONS

Relieving heat accumulation by mild effect.

Mild cases of excess syndrome of yangming-fu organ, manifested as delirium, tidal fever, constipation, distension and fullness in the chest and abdomen, yellow shriveled tongue coating, smooth and swift pulse as well as the onset of dysentery with distending abdominal pain or epigastric fullness, tenesmus.

Minor Decoction for Strengthening
the Middle-warmer
(Xiao jian zhong tang)

INGREDIENTS

Radix Paconiae	18g
Ramulus Cinnamomi	9g
Radix Glycyrrhizae	6g
Rhizoma Zingiberis Recens	10g
Fructus Ziziphi Jujubae	4 pcs
Saccharum Granorum	30g

The decoction is prepared by decocting all the drugs but the last one, filtering out the residue, and adding Saccharum Granorum into the already-decocted solution. It should be taken warm.

INDICATIONS

Warming the middle-warmer, tonifying deficiency and relieving spasm and pain. Abdominal pain due to cold of deficiency type, marked by abdominal pain which can be relieved by warming and pressing; or consumptive diseases manifested by palpitation, restlessness, pale complexion, whitish coating of the tongue, thready, taut and weak pulse; or fever due to yang-deficiency.

Contraindicated in cases with hyperactivity of pathogenic fire due to yin-deficiency. Not administered to those suffering from vomiting since the sweet flavor of the drugs may induce vomiting.

INTERPRETATION

The last ingredient in the recipe, which is dominant is dosage, is referred to as a principal drug because its sweet taste and warm nature facilitates its effect on the splcen, and it is able to replenish the spleen-qi and nourish the spleen-yin, having the functions not only in warming the middle-warmer and restoring qi but also in regulating the internal organs and relieving spasm. Both Peony root and Cinnamon twig play the part of an assistant drug: the former, sour in flavour and slightly cold in nature, has the function of replenishing yin-blood to relieve spasm and pain, and the latter, pungent in flavour and warm in narure, is effective for supporting yang-qi. The combined administration of the above two drugs- one warm in nature and beneficial to yang and the other cold and beneficial to yin-helps to regulate ying and wei, yin and yang. The rest are used together as adjuvant and guiding drugs. No. 4 is used to replenish wei-yang . No. 5 is used to tonify ying-yin and strengthen the spleen and stomach, and NO. 3 to regulate the middle-warmer and replenish qi. Upon analysis, recipe is this recipe for warming the middle-warmer, tonifying qi and relieving spasm and pain.

Studies in recent years have confirmed that this recipe possesses the efficacies in relieving spasm, alleviating pain, promoting blood circulation, strengthening digestion and absorption, promoting the healing of ulcers, nourishing the body, consolidating the constitution, etc.

Minor Decoction of Bupleurum
(Xiao chai hu tang)

INGREDIENTS

Radix Bupleuri	12g
Radix Scutellariae	9g
Rhizoma Pinelliae	9g
Rhizoma Zingiberis Recens	9g
Radix Ginseng	6g
Fructus Ziziphi Jujubae	4 pcs
Radix Glycyrrhizae Praeparata	5g

INDICATIONS

Treating shaoyang disease by mediation. Shaoyang disease with the pathogenic factors located neither in the exterior nor in the interipr but in between marked by alternate attacks of chills and fever, fullness in the chest, hypochondriac discomfort, anorexia, dysphoria, retching, bitterness in the mouth, dry throat, dizziness, thin and white fur of the tobngue and stringy pulse, or exogenous febrile diseases occurring in women belonging to invasion of the blood chamber by pathogenic heat.

The common cold, malaria, infection of biliary tract, hepatitis, pleuritis, chronic gastritis, indigestion, mastosis, intercostal neuralgia, neurosis and AIDS marked by the symptoms of shaoyang disease can be treated by the modified recipe.

Patients with syndromes such as upper excess with lower deficiency, or excess of liver-fire, hyperactivity of the liver-yang, haematemesis due to deficiency of yin are forbidden to use the recipe.

INTERPRETATION

Bupleurum root as a principal drug, dispels the pathogenic factor located in the half exterior by driving it out. Scutellaria root clears out stagnated heat located in the half interior by clearing away it thoroughly as an assistant drug. The combined use of the two drugs, one for dispelling pathogen, and the other for clearing away stagnated heat, removes pathogenic factors from shaoyang channels. Pinellia tuber and Fresh ginger regulate the function of the stomach and lower the adverse flow of qi. Ginseng and Chinese dates invigorate qi and strengthen the middle-warmer. Prepared licorice root coordinates the actions of various drugs in the recipe. The drugs from No. 3 to No. 7 act as adjuvant and guiding drugs.

Modern researches have proved that the recipe has some effects of inhibiting bacteria, viruses and leptospira, reliecing the reaction of the human body to the invaded pathogen, and remarkably allaying fever and resisting inflammation. In addition, the recipe also has the effects of promoting digestion, preventing vomiting, expelling phlegm, relieving ecugh, protecting the liver, normalizing the functioning of the gallbaldder and tranquilizing the mind.

Ophiopogon Decoction
(Mai men dong tang)

INGREDIENTS

Radix Ophiopogonis	60g
Rhizoma Pineliae	9g
Radix Ginseng	6g
Radix Glycyrrhizae	4g
Oryza Glutinosae	6g
Fructus Ziziphi Jujubae	3 pcs

Decocted in water for oral administration.

INDICATIONS

Nourishing the lung and the stomach, loweing the adverse flow of qi and regulating the stomach.

Consumptive lung disease marked by cough, whitish frothy sputum, shortness of breath, dryness of the mouth and pharynx, this, dryness of the tongue red in colour with little fur and weak and rapid pulse.

Chronic bronchitis, chronic pharyngitis, pulmonary tuberculosis, bronchiectasis, chronic gastritis, atrophic gastritis, and epidemic febrile diseases in the recover stage marked by deficiency of both the stomach-qi and stomach-yin can be treated by the modified recipe.

The recipe is contraindicated in patients with consumptive lung disease belonging to tfhe cold of insufficiency type.

INTERPRETATION

Lilyturf root in the recipe, used in large dosage as a principal drug, nourishes the lung-yin and stomach-yin and clears away the fire of deficiency type. Pinellia tuber is aimed at lowering the adverse flow of qi to resolve phlegm, as an assistant drug. In spite of its dry nature when it is used in combination with a large dosage of Lilyturf root its dry nature is reduced but its effect of lowering the adverse flow of qi remained. It also enables Lilyturf root to keep its tonic effect and lose its greasy nature. Ginseng replenishes and restores the middle-warmer qi. When it is used in combination with Lilyturf root, its effects of invigorating qi and producing body fluids can be strengthened. Glutinous rice, Chinese-dates and licorice root as adjuvant and guiding drugs, tonify the spleen and benefit the stomach.

Modern researches have proved that the recipe has the effects of nourishing and mostening the human body, relieving cough and eliminating phlegm.

Oriental Wormwood Decoction
(Yin chen hao tang)

INGREDIENTS

Herba artemisiae Capillaris	30g
Fructus gardenia	15g
Radix et Rhizoma Rhei	9g

Decocted in water for oral administration.

INDICATIONS

Clearing away heat and eliminating dampness to treat jaundice. Jaundice dur to damp-heat characterized by bright yellow coloration of the skin and eyes, slight fullness sensation in the abdomen, thirst, disturbance in urination, yellow and greasy tongue fur and deep and rapid pulse.

Patients with acute infectious icteric hepatitis, cholecystitis, cholelithiasis and acute pancreatitis marked by the syndrome of jaundice due to damp-heat can be treated by the modified recipe.

The recipe is contraindicated in patients with jaundice of yin type.

INTERPRETATION

Oriental wormwood in the recipe is used in large dosage as a principal drug to clear away heat and dampness for the treatment of jaundice. Capejasmine fruit guides dampness and heat downward and eliminates dampness and heat through urination, as an assistant drug. Rhubarb purges away heat, removes blood stasis and relieves constipation, as an adjuvant drug.

Modern researches have proved that the recipe is effective in normalizing the function of the gallbladder, nourishing the liver, allaying fever, relieving inflammation and inducing diuresis and has, in addition, the purgative, antibacterial, antiviral and bleeding-arresting effects.

Peony Decoction
(Shao yao tang)

INGREDIENTS

Radix Paeoniae	15g
Radix Angelicae Sinensis	9g
Rhizoma Coptidis	9g
Semen Arecae	5g
Radix Aucklandiae	5g
Radix Glycyrrhizae	5g
Radix et Rhizoma Rhei	9g
Radix Scutellariae	9g
Cortex Cinnamomi	5g

All the ingredients should be decocted in water for oral administration.

INDICATIONS

Clearing away damp-heat and toxic material and regulating qi and blood.

Diarrhea or dysentery due to damp-heat pathogen marked by abdominal pain, pus and blood in the stool, tenesmus, burning sensation in the anus, scanty deepcoloured urine, yellow greasy coating of the tongue, etc.

The recipe can be modified to treat acute enteritis, bacillary dysentery and other conditions indicative of damp-heat in the large intestine.

It is not advisable for cases with external syndromes at the onset of dysentery nor for those suffering from chronic dysentery or deficiency-cold dysentery.

INTERPRETATION

Peony root as a principal drug, is administered in larger dosage to regulate qi and blood for the treatment of abdominal pain and tenesmus caused by dysentery. Coptis root, Rhubarb and Scutellaria root share the effects of clearing away heat and removing toxic materials. chinese angelica root and Cinnamon bark give the effects of regulating the ying and promoting circulation of blood. Areca seed and Aucklandia root are indicated for promoting the flow of qi and removing stagnancy. Liquorice root coordinates various effects of all the drugs in the recipe.

Modern researches have confirmed the effects of this recipe in resisting bacteria, subduing inflammation, and relieving spasm and pain.

Peptic Powder
(Ping wei san)

INGREDIENTS

Rhizoma Atractylodis	15g
Cortex Magnoliae Officinalis	9g
Pericarpium Citri Reticulatae	9g
Radix Glycyrrhizae	4g

Grind the above drugs into fine powder. Take 3 to 5 grams each time with the decoction of fresh ginger and chinese-dates; or decoct them in water for oral adiministration.

INDICATIONS

Drying dampness and strengthening the spleen, promoting the circulation of qi and regulating the stomach. Stagnancy of dampness in the stomach and spleen marked by feeling of fullness in the abdomen, nausea, vomiting, eructation, acid regurgitation, white, greasy and thick tongue fur and slow pulse.

Acute gastroenteritis, catarrhal gastritis, gastrointestinal neurosis and acute indigestion marked by the syndrome of stagnancy of dampness in the stomach and spleen can be treated by the modified recipe.

The recipe, bitter in taste, pungent in flavor, warm and dry in nature, tends to consume yin and blood, There-fore, it is contraindicated in patients suffering from deficiency of the spleen without dampness or patients with deficiency-yin marked by red tongue with little fur, bitter taste in the mouth with thirst or rapid pulse.

INTERPRETATION

Atractylodes rhizome used in large dosage as a principal drug, dispels dampness to promote the function of the spleen. Magnolia bark promotes the circulation of qi and eliminates dampness to relieve distension and fullness in the abdomen, acting as an assistant drug. Tangerine peel regulates qi and eliminates dampness, as an adjuvant drug. Licorice root sweet in taste and mild in nature, regulates the stomach and coordinates the effects of the other drugs in the recipe. Fresh ginger and Chinese-dates regulate the functions of the spleen and the stomach.

Modern researches have proved that the recipe has the effects of regulating gastrointestinal function and eliminating excessive water from the body.

Pill for Invigorating Spleen
(Jian pi wan)

INGREDIENTS

Rhizoma Atractylodis Macrocephalae (parched)	75g
Radix Aucklandiae (to be ground seperately from others)	22g
Rhizoma Coptidis (wine-parched)	22g
Radix Glycyrrhizae	22g
Poria	60g
Radix Ginseng	45g
Massa Fermentata Medicinalis (parched)	30g
Pericarpium Citri Reticulatae	30g
Fructus Amoni	30g
Fructus Hordei Germinatus (parched)	30g
Fructus Crataegi	30g
Rhizoma Dioscoreae	30g

Semen Myristicae (floured wrapped in paper and beaten by a hand mallet so as to get rid of its oil) 30g

Make paste pills or make pills with water. The pills are to be tadken 6-9 grams each time with warm boiled water twice a day.

INDICATIONS

Strengthening the spleen and regulating the stomach, pronoting digestion and arresting diarrhea. Retention of food dur to deficiency of the spleen marked by poor appetite, indigestion, distention and fullness in the stomach and abdomen, loose bowels, greasy coating of the tongue, and feeble pulse.

The modification of the recipe is advisable for the above syndrome as seen in cases such as chronic enteritis, disturbance of intestinal function, irritable colon, etc.

It is not fit for those with tetention of food brought about by improper eating, overeating and overdrinking.

INTERPRETATION

In the recipe, Nos. 1, 4, 5 and 6 are considered as four noble ingredients which can provide the effect of reinforcing qi and the spleen, of which bighead atractylodes rhizome and Poria are inhibited in larger dosage to reinforce mainly the spleen, excrete dampness and stop diarrhea. To assist the four ingredients, the last two ingredients are administered to strengthen the efficacies in reinforcing the spleen and stopping the diarrhea. Nos. 7, 10 and 11 are used to promote digestion and remove stangated food, Nos, 8, and 9 to regulate qi and the stomach; coptis root clear away heat and dampness.

As modern researches have confirmed, this recipe has the efficacies in adjusting intestinal function, promoting digestion, relieving inflammation, resisting bacteria, etc.

Pill for Relieving Stagnancy
(Yue ju wan)

INGREDIENTS

Rhizoma Cyperi

Rhizoma Ligustici Chuanxiong

Rhizoma Atractylodis

Fructus Garaeniae

Massa Fermentata Medicinalis

The dose of the ingredients is equal in amount

Grind the above-mentioned ingredients into fine powder first, and then make pills with water. Take 6 to 9 grams each time.

INDICATIONS

Promoting the circulation of qi to relieve the stagnation. Syndrome of sic kinds of stagnations marked by oppressed sensation and feeling of stufffiness in the chest, epigastric distesion and pain, gastric discomfort with acid reurgitation, indigestion, eructation, vomiting and nausea, white and greasy fur of the tongue, taut pulse.

Gastrointestinal neurosis, gastroduodenal ulcer, chronic gastritis, infectious hepatitis, cholecystitis, cholelithiasis, intercostal neuralgia, dysmenorrhea and others marked by symptoms of six kinds of stagnations can be treated by the modified recipe.

This recipe is indicated only for the stagnancies belonging to excess syndromes. Stagnancies associated with deficiency type should not be treated only with this recipe.

INTERPRETATION

Nutgrass flatsedge rhizome in the recipe is used as a principal drug to deal with stagnancy of qi by promoting the circulation of qi. Chuanxiong rhizome promotes the circulation of qi and blood to treat stagnancy of blood. Atractylodes rhizome can treat stagnancy of dampness by reinforcing the spleen. Capejasmine fruit can treat stagnancy of fire by clearing away pathogenic heat and purging pathogenic fire. Medicated laeaven can treat stagnancy of food by promoting digestion and normalizing the function of the stomach. All the abovementioned drugs are used as assistant drugs. As the stagnancy of phlegm is mainly caused by spleen-dampness and associated with stagnancy of qi, fire and food, and it can be cleared away when the other various stagnacies are removed.

Modern studies have proved that this recipe has the effects of tranquilizing the mind, alleviating pain, promoting digestion, and relieving spasm of uterine smooth muscle.

Pill for Relieving
the distention of Middle Jiao
(Zhong man fen xiao wan)

INGREDIENTS

Cortex Magnoliae Officinalis (prepared with ginger)	12g
Rhizoma Atractylodis Macrocephalae	6g
Radix Codonopsis Pilosulae	6g
Rhizoma Curcumae Longae	6g
Rhizoma Zingiberis	6g
Rhizoma Alismatis	6g
Exocarpium Citri Grandis	6g
Rhizoma Anemarrhenae	6g
Polyporus Umbellatus	10g
Poria	10g
Radix Scutellariae	10g
Rhizoma Coptidis	10g
Rhizoma Pinelliae	10g
Fructus Aurantii Immaturus (fried)	10g
Radix glycyrrhizae Praeparata	3g
Fructus Amomi	3g

ACTION

Activating the spleen and vital energy, clearing away heat and promoting diuresis; mainly for cases with retention of dampness-heat and accumulation of fluid, which manifest as abdominal fullness and pain, irritability, bitter taste in the mouth, thirst but unwilling to drink, oliguria with reddish urine, constipation, yellow and greasy fur on the tongue, wiry and rapid pulse.

INDICATIONS

1. For cases of jaundice accompanied with fatigue, feeling of fullness over the chest and abdomen, poor appetite, nausea, loose stools, yellow and greasy fur on the tongue, soft and floating, slow pulse, which are attributive to the dysfunction of spleen and the stagnation of dampness-heat (predominantly dampness), omit Glycyrrhizae and apply Herba Artemisiaw Scopariae instead of Ane-

marrhenae to enhance the diuretic and anti-icteric effects.

2. For cases of leucorrhagia with a large amount of yellow-whitish, thick foul discharge, accompanied with dizziness, fatigue, abdominal fullness, poor appetite, yellow and greasy fur on the tongue, wiry and smooth pulse, which are attributive to the dysfunction of spleen and downward attack of dampness-heat (predominantly dampness), the doses of Atractylodis Macrocephalae and Poria in the prescritpion should be increased.

3. Also applicable to cases of cirrhosis of liver and tuberculous peritonitis with ascites, icterus infectious hepatitis and cholecystitis with jaundice, endometritis and trichomonas vagintis with leucorrhagia, which are attributive to dysfunction of spleen and downward attack of dampness-heat.

INTERPRETATION

Magnoliae Officinalis, Aurantii Immarturus, Curcumae Longae have the effects of activating circulation of vital energy and relieving fullness. Zingiberis and Pinelliae serve to eliminate dampness-heat when they are used together with Coptidis. Alismatis and Polyporus Umbellatus promote diuresis. Citri Grandis and Amomi, when used together with Scutellariae, Atractylodis Macrocephalae, Codonopsis Pilosulae and Glycyrrhizae serve to activate the spleen and stomach and to disperse phlegm-dampness. In sum, the prescription can get rid of dampness-heat and excessive fluid from the spleen and stomach.

Pill of Aucklandiae and Arecae
(Mu xiang bing lang wan)

INGREDIENTS

Radix Aucklandiae	12g
Semen Arecae	12g
Radix et Rhizoma Rhei	12g
Rhizoma Coptidis(fried with bran)	10g
Cortex Phellodendri	10g
Rhizoma Cyperi	10g
Semen Pharbitidis	6g
Pericarpium Citri Reticulatae Viride	6g

Pericarpium Citri Reticulatae	3g
Rhizoma Zedoariae	3g
Rhizoma Zingiberis Recens	3 pcs

ACTION

Promoting circulation of vital energy, eliminating stagnancy of food and clearing away heat evil; mainly for cases due to stagnation of indigestive foods and functional disorder of intestines, manifested as abdominal pain and fullness, diffficulty in urination and defecation, yellow and greasy fur on the tongue, sunken and solid pulse.

INDICATION

1. For cases of dysentery attributive to dampness-heat accompanied with indigestion, manifested as difficulty in defecation, discharge of reddish or whitish stools, burning sensation over the anus, abdominal distending pain, yellow and greasy fur on the tongue and smooth pulse, omit Zedoariae and Pharbitidis from this prescription and add Radix Pulsatillae.

2. Also applicable to cases of cirrhotic ascites, chronic nephritis, tuyberculous peritonitis, ets. , marked by abdominal fullness, defficulty in urination and defecation, and cases of bacillary dysentery, acute cnteritis, etc. , marked by dearrhea, which are attributive to stagnation of indigestive foods with transporting disorder of intestine or production of dampness-heat evil.

INTERPRETATION

Aucklandiae and Arecae serve as the principal drugs for promoting the circulation of vital energy and eliminating stagnancy of food, Cyperi, Citri Reticulatae Viride, Citri Reticulatae, Zingiberis Recens and Zedoariae are applied for regulating the activities of liver, spleen, intestine and stomach, and restoring their transporting function. Coptidis and Phellodendri are for clearing away heat evil from the intestine and stomach, Rhei for loosing the bowel and Pharbitidis for promoting diuresis. In summary, this is a representative prescription for difficulty in urination and defecation due to stagnation of indigestive foods with production of heat evil while the healthy energy is not yet deficient. Most of its components are acrid and aromatic in nature, with action of activating the circulation of vital energy.

Pill of Four Miraculous Drugs
(Si shen wan)

INGREDIENTS

Semen Myristicae	60g
Fructus Psoralese	120g
Fructus Schisandrae	60g
Fructus Evodiae	30g

Add 240 grams of fresh ginger and 100 pieces of Chinese-dates to the above-mentioned grugs. Grind them into powder tŏ make pills for oral administration. Take 9 to 12 grams each time before going to bed with light salty water or warm boiled water.

INDICATIONS

Warming and tonifying the spleen and kidney to relieve diarrhea with astringency. Diarrhea due to deficiency of the kidney-yang manifested as diarrhea before dawn, anorexia, loose stools with undigested food, abdominal pain, lumbago, coldness of the limbs, listlessness, pale tongue with whitish fur, and deep, slow and feeble pulse.

Patients with chronic enteritis, intestinal tuberculosis, ulcerative inflammation of large intestine and other chronic diseases, or old people, manifested by diarrhea before dawn due to yang-deficiency of the spleen and kidney can be treated by the modified recipe.

The recipe is contraindicated in the patients with diarrhea due to indigestion ar accumulation of heat in the stomach and intestine.

INTERPRETATION

Psoralea fruit with a pungent flavor, bitter taste, warm nature and having the effect of invigoration the gate of life (kidney-yang), is an important drug for strengthening physiological fire (motive force of life) and replenishing earth (the spleen), used as a principal drug. Nutmeg warms the spleen and kidney and relieves diarrhea with astringency, and Evodia fruit warms the spleen and stomach to dispel cold and dampness, both acting as assistant drugs. Magnolia vine fruit is a swrm-natured and astringent drug, fresh ginger dispels dampness and promotes the flow of water and chinese-dates nourishes the spleen and stomach.

they are all used as adjuvant and guiding drugs.

.Modern researches have proved that the recipe has the effects of protecting the mucosa of stomach and intestine, arresting diarrhea and allergic reaction.

Pill of Immature Bitter
Orange for Removing Stagnancy
(Zhi shi dao zhi wan)

INGREDIENTS

Radix et Rhizoma Rhei	30g
Fructus Aurantii Immaturus	15g
Massa Fermentata Medicinalis	15g
Poria	9g
Radix Scutellariae	9g
Rhizoma Coptidis	9g
Rhizoma Atractylodis Macrocephalae	9g
Rhizoma Allismatis	6g

ACTION

The drugs are ground into particles and then made into pills by refining powder with water, to be taken 6-9g each time with warm boiled water, twice a day. The drugs may also be decocted in water for oral administration. The dosage is reduced in proportion as the original recipe.

INDICATIONS

Promoting digestion to remove stagnated food and eliminating dampness-heat.

Syndrome due to stagnated food and dampness-heat manifested as epigastric distress and fullness, dysentery and diarrhea, or constipation, scanty and deep-coloured urine, yellow and greasy coating of the tongue and slow and vigorous pulse.

Moreover, other diseases such as acute indigestion, gastroenteritis, bacterial diarrhea and others that indicate stagnancy of food and dampness-heat in the spleen and stomach may be treated with the modified recipe.

Inadvisable for patients with stagnated food due to deficiency of the spleen.

INTERPRETATION

In the recipe, Rhubarb root dominates in dosage and acts as the principal drug used to clean up the stagnancy of food. Immature bitter orange as an assistant drug, promotes the flow of qi and scatters food accumulation. The rest all share the role of adjuvant and guiding drugs, of which, Scutellaria root and Coptis root both contribute their effort in removing heat-dampness, and arresting dysentery; Poria and Oriental water plantain rhizome devote in combination their effects in inducing diuresis, excreting dampness and arresting diarrhea, and big-head atractylodes rhizome plays its part in strengthening the spleen and removing dampness.

As modern researches have confirmed, this recipe possesses the efficacies in promoting peristalsis of the stomach and intestines, assisting in digestion and absorption, and functions in arresting diarrhea, inducing diuresis, relieving inflammation, resisting bacteria and others by purgation.

Pill of Sanguisorbae
(Di gu wan)

INGREDIENTS

Radix Sanguisorbae (fried)	15g
Radix Angelicae Sinensis (fried)	10g
Colla Corii Asini (fried with glutinous rice)	10g
Rhizoma coptidis	10g
Fructus Chebulae (fried)	10g
Fructus Mume (nut removed)	10g
Radix Aucklandiae	6g

ACTION

Cooling blood, removing toxic material, stopping bleeding and diarrhea; mainly for cases of diarrhea attributive to attack of dampness-heat and consumption of yin-blood, which are manifested as discharge of purplish, bloody and mucous stool, tenesmus, continuous abdominal pain general debility, fatigue, red and uncoated tongue, sunken and small. rapid pulse, etc.

INDICATIONS

1. Applicable to cases of hemorrhoidal bleeding with bitter mouth, dry throat, red and uncoated tongue, which are attributive to hyperactivity of heat in xuefen and deficiency of ying-yin.

2. Also applicable to cases of chronic bacillary dysentery, amebic dysentery, chronic colitis, intestinal tuberculosis, etc., which are attributive to retention of dampness-heat(predominantly heat) and consumption of yin-blood.

INTERPRETATION

Sanguisorbae serves to clear away heat from xuefen and also has an astringing and hemotatic effect; while Coptidis clears away heat from qifen and also a dampness-drying and antidysenteric effect. when used together they are superior for dysentery with hyperactivity of heat in xuefen and complicated by attack of dampness. Colla Corii Asini can not only nourish yin and tonify blood but also stop bleeding, and fortify yin and relieve dysentery when used together with Coptidis. The above three drugs serve as the prinicipal drugs in this prescription. Angelicae Sinensis regulates ying and promtes blood circulation, and can relieve the discharge of purulent and bloody stools. Aucklandiae promotes circulation of vital energy and dredges stagnation, and can relieve tenesmus. Mune and Chebulae have the effect of astringing the intestines to decrease bowel movement, and are used for the treatment of chronic dysentery with consumption of yin-blood. But it should be emphasized that the therapy of cooling blood and eliminating toxic material is the main treatment for those cases, otherwise, the evil may be ratained if only the astringing therapy is applied.

Pill of Three Drugs for Emergency
(San wu bei ji wan)

INGREDIENTS

    Radix et Rhizoam Rhei

    Fructus Crotonis (coat and embryo discarded, then ground)

    Rhizoma Zingiberis, āā equal amount

Ground into powder and prepared as pills, to be taken 0. 5-1. 5g each time.

ACTION

Eliminating the stagnated cold, promoting bowel movement and alleviating pain; mainly for cases attributive to stagnation of cold and sluggishness of vital energy, which manifest as sudden onset of stabbing pain over the precordial area and abdomen, constipation, or even coma, cold limbs, shortness of breath and lockjaw, turbid and greasy fur on the tongue, sunken and tense or sunken and slow pulse.

INDICATIONS

1. The prescription is a potent purgative, in which Fructus Crotonis is poisonous. It should be only applied in case of emergency and when the patient is still strong enough.

2. If diarrhea occurs too frequently after taking the decoction, cold porridge should be given.

3. Applicable to cases of ascites with dyspnea, oliguria, constipation, white and greasy fur, sunken and solid pulse, when the patient is still strong.

4. Also applicable to cases of intestinal obstruction, food poisoning (after 3-4 hours), cirrhosis of liver, liver cancer, etc., which are attributive to accumulation of cold in the interior.

INTERPRETATION

Crotonis is a potent drug for eliminating cold from the gastrointestines and purging the stagnation of the digestivetract. Zingiberis has the effect of warming middle jiao and help Crotonis to eliminate cold. Rhei is used as a purgative to relieve the stagnation of intenstines. The bitter-cold nature of Rhei is counteracted by Zingiberis and Crotonis. The combination of thesr three drugs exerts a strong effect for the emergency cases with cold stagnation.

Pill with Immature Bitter Orange for
Disintegrating Masses and Relieving Stuffiness
(Zhi shi xiao pi wan)

INGREDIENTS

Rhizoma Zingiberis	3g
Radix Glycyrrhizae Praeparata	6g
Fructus Hordei Germinatus	6g
Poria	6g

Rhizoma Atractylodis Macrocephalae	6g
Rhizoma Pinelliae	9g
Radix Ginseng	9g
Cortex Magnoliae Officinalis	12g
Fructus Aurantii Immaturus	15g
Cortex Phellodendri	15g

Make water-pills or make paste pills. The pills are to be taken 6-9 grams each time with warm boiled water, twice a day.

INDICATION

Disintegrating masses and relieving distention and fullness, strengthening the spleen and regulating the stomach. Masses or distension and fullness due to deficiency of the spleen marked by epigastric masses, distension and fullness, loss of appetite, general debility, or distension and fullness in the chest and hypochondrium accompanied by poor appetite, indigestion difficult bowel movement, greasy coating of the tongue and slippery pulse.

The modified recipe is advisable for the above syndrome occurring in cases of chronic gastritis and chronic diarrhea.

INTERPRETATION

In the recipe, Immature bitter orange is referred to as a principal drug, giving the effects of promoting the flow of qi and disintegrating masses. Acting as an assistant drug, Prepared magnolia bark has the same effect as immature bitter orange and is therefore used to reinforce the effect of the principal drug. The combination of the above two drugs results in strengthening the effect of relieving distension and fullness. The last drug has the effects of clearing up heat and removing dampness to disintegrate masses. Medicated leaven of pinellia tuber, pungent and warm in property, has the effects of removing dampness and regulating the stomach. And dried ginger is capable of warming the stomach and spleen to dispel cold. Ginseng is able to strengthen the body resistance and reinforce the spleen, poria and bighead atractylodes rhizome both able to strengthen the spleen and remove dampness, medicated leaven of germinated barley able to promote the digestion and regulate the stomach, and prepared licorice root is used as the temper of all the drugs in the recipe.

Powder for Clearing Stomach-heat
(Qing wei san)

INGREDIENTS

Radix Rehmanniae	12g
Radix Angelicae Sinensis	6g
Cortex Moutan Radicis	9g
Rhizoma Coptidis	3g
Rhizoma Cimicifugae	6g

Decocted in water, for oral administration.

INDICATIONS

Clearing stomach-heat and removing heat from the blood. Stagnation of heat in the stomach marked by headache radiated by toothache, feverish cheeks, aversion to heat with predilection for cold, ulceration in the gum, or gingival atrophy with oozing of bloody fluid and pus, or swelling and soreness of the tongue, lips and cheeks, or hot and foul breath, dryness of mouth and tongue, reddened tongue with yellow coating, and slippery strong and rapid pulse.

The recipe can be modified to deal with periodontitis, stomatitis, gingival pustular swelling, glossitis and gastritis indicative of stomach-heat.

It is not fit for patients with toothache of wind-cold type and toothache caused by hyperactivity of fire due to yin deficiency.

INTERPRETATION

In the recipe. coptis root being bitter in taste and cold in nature, is used as a principal drug, providing the effect of clearnig the fire in heart and stomach. Dried rehmannia root and moutan bark are used in combination as assistant drugs; the former possessing the effect of removing heat from the blood and nourishing yin and the latter having the function of removing heat from the blood, reducing pathogenic heat. Chinese angelica as an adjuvant drug, has the effects of nourishing the blood, promoting blood circulation and subduing swelling and alleviating pain. Cimicifuga rhizome can dispel pathogenic fire and remove toxic substances. The coordination of various drugs results in clearing stomach-heat and removing pathogenic heat from the blood.

Modern researches have proved that the recipe possesses the efficacies of resisting bacteria, subduing inflammation, arresting bleeding, bringing down fever, tranquilizing the mind, relieving pain and promoting blood circulation.

Powder for Treating Cold Limbs
(Si ni san)

INGREDIENTS

Radix Bupleuri	6g
Radix Paeoniae Alba	9g
Fructus Aurantii Immaturus	6g
Radix Glycyrrhizae Praeparata	6g

All the above drugs are decocted in water for oral administration.

INDICATIONS

Dispersing pathogens and alleviating mental depression, soothing the liver and regulating the spleen. Cold limbs due to the internal depressed yang-qi which fails to reach the distal parts of limbs, or epigastric distension and distress, diarrhea with tenesmus and abdominal pain caused by stagnation of the livet-qi and the accumulation of the spleen-qi, white fur of the tongue and stringy pulse.

Patients with chronic hepatitis, cholecystitis, cholelithiasis, pancreatitis, neuralgia intercostalis and gastroneurosis marked by the symptoms of stagnation of liver-qi and the accumulation of the spleen-qi can be treated by the modified recipe.

Since it is indicated for cold limbs due to excess of heat which is caused by stagnation of yang-qi, the recipe is contraindicated in patients with cold limbs of other types.

INTERPRETATION

Bupleurum root soothes the liver, regulates the circulation of qi and normalizes the functional activities of qi to render pathogenic heat out of the human body. White peony root nourishes the liver, relieves spasm and replenishes yin, so that pathogenic heat is removed from the body without impairing yin. Fruit of immature citron purges stagnation from the spleen. Prepared licorice root coordinates the effects of all the drugs in the recipe and can relieve spasm and pain in combination with white peony root.

Modern researches have proved that the recipe has the effects of tranquilizing the mind, relieving spasm and pain, allaying fever and resisting bacteria. In addition, it is also very effective in treating hepatic injury.

Powder of Agastachis for Restoring Healthy Energy
(Huo xiang zheng qi San)

INGREDIENTS

Pericarpium Arecae	30g
Radix Angelicae Dahuricae	30g
Folium Perillae	30g
Poria	30g
Rhizoma Pinelliae	60g
Rhizoma Atractylodis Macrocephalae	60g
Perticarpium Citri Reticulatae	60g
Cortex Magnoliae Officinalis(bark removed, ginger-juice-fried)	
	60g
Radix Platycodi	60g
Herba Agastachis	90g
Radix Glycyrrhizae Praeparata	75g

Grind the drugs into fine powder. Take 6 grams each time with decoction of fresh ginger and Chinese-dates, or decoct them in water for oral administration.

INDICATIONS

Relieving exterior syndrome, eliminating dampness and regulating qi and the stomach. Vomiting and diarrhea due to exterior cold with interior dampness marked by chills, fever, headache, fullness sensation and oppressed feeling in the chest and abdomen, vomiting, diarrhea, borborygmus and abdominal pain, and thick and greasy tongue fur.

The common cold of gastrointestinal type, influenza, acute gastroenteritis, gastroduodenal ulcer, chronic colitis, food poisoning, epidemic parotitis and other diseases belonging to exterior cold with endogenous can be treated with the modified recipe.

Since mainly composed of pungent, aromatic, warmnatured and desiccant drugs, the recipe is contraindicated in patients with excessive fire due to deficiency of yin. In addition, patients with thirst and yellow and greasy tongue fur should use the recipe with great care.

When used in the form of decoction, the drugs should be decocted for a shorter time to prevent the decrease in effect.

INTERPRETATION

Wrinkled gianthyssop is administered in large dosage as a principal drug. It can not only dispel wind-cold but also expel the turbid pathogen and regulate the stomach to arrest vomiting; meanwhile it can send up the lucid qi and send down the turbid, clear away summer-heat and filthy pathogens. Leaf of purple perilla and Dahurian angelica root, effective in dispersing exopathogens, assist Wrinkled gianthyssop in dispersing wind and cold from the body surface and eliminate dampness concurrently by means of its aroma. Pinellia tuber and Tangerine peel dry dampness and regulate the stomach, lower the adverse flow of qi to arrest vomiting. Bighead atractylodes rhizoma and Tuckahoe strengthen the spleen and the stomach and regulate the middle-warmer to arrest diarrhea. Shell of areca nut and Magnolia bark promote the circulation of qi, dispel dampness, regulate the middle-warmer to relieve fullness sensation in the abdomen. Root of balloon-flower, which can facilitate the flow of the lung-qi and relieve fullness in the chest and hypochondrium, is helpful in dispersing dampness as well as in relieving the exterior syndrome. Fresh ginger, Chinese-dates and Prepared licorice root regulate the functions of the spleen and the stomach.

Modern researches have proved that the recipe has better effects of regulating gastrointestinal function, arresting vomiting and diarrhea and reinforcing the stomach; meanwhile, it has the effects of inducing diaphoresis, allaying fever, relieving pain, resisting bacteria and virus, eliminating phlegm, relieving cough, inducing diuresis.

Powder of Bupleuri for Dispersing
the Depressed Liver-energy
(Chai hu shu gan san)

INGREDIENT

Radix Bupleuri	10g
Fructus Aurantii	10g
Rhizoma Ligustici Chuanxiong	10g
Exocarpium Citri Grandis	10g
Rhizoma Cyperi	10g
Radix Paeoniae Alba	15g
Radix Glycyrrhizae Praeparata	6g

ACTION

Dispersing the stagnated liver-energy, regulating vital energy, activating blood circulation and relieving pain; mainly for cases due to stagnation of liver-energy and vital energy manifested as fullness of breast, hypochondriac pain, or dysmenorrhea, or stomachache, and for cases due to stagnation of liver and gall-bladder heat manifested as alternating episodes of chills and fever.

INDICATION

1. This prescription and Powder for Treating Yang Exhaustion both have the similar action and indication, but the former, owning to the action of Bupleuri, has a stronger effect on dispersing the stagnated liver-energy, regulating the vital and activating blood circulation. It is frequently applied for the cases of menoxenia or distending pain of the breast.

2. For cases with distending pain of the breast, add Radix Salviae Miltiorrhizae and Fructus Hordei Germinatus(30 g) to disperse the stagnated liver-energy and promote blood circulation; for cases with alternating episodes of chills and fever, omit Ligustici Chuanxiong and add Radix Scutellariae and Herba Artemisiae Annuae to clear away the gallbladder heat.

3. Also applicable to cases of pleurisy, cholecystitis, mastitis, hyperplasea of mammary gland, etc. , which are attributive to stagnation of liver-energy and vital energy.

INTERPRETATION

This prescription is formed on the basis of Decoction for Treating Yang Exhaustion, by using Aurantii instead of Aurantii Immaturus and adding Cyperi, Citri Grandis, Ligustici Chuanxiong. Bupleuri and Ligustci Chuanxiong have the effect of dreding the stagnation of blood in the liver channel; Cyperi and Aurantii Immaturus has the effect of dredging the stagnation of vital energy in the liver channel; Paeoniae Alba and Glycyrrhizae has the effects of softening the liver and preventing the above drugs from damaging yin. All the above used together serve to disperse the stagnated liver-energy, soften the liver and promote the circulation of vital energy and blood.

Powder of Five Drugs with Poria
(Wu ling san)

INGREDIENTS

Polyporus Umbellatus	9g
Rhizoma Alismatis	15g
Rhizoma Atractylodis Macrocephalae	9g
Poria	9g
Ramulus Cinnamomi	6g

All the drugs should be made into pulvis and taken 3 to 6 grams each time, or decocted in water for oral administration.

INDICATIONS

Removing dampness by promoting diuresis and warming yang to promote the functions of qi.

Syndrome of fluid retention within the body marked by headache, fever, thirst with vomiting after drinking water, disturbance in urination, white greasy fur or white and thick fur and floating pulse; or edema, diarrhea, fluid-retention syndrome, dizziness and a feeling of palpitation in the lower abdomen.

Acute gastroenteritis, cyclic vomiting, pseudocholera, urticaria of cold type, initial stage of acute nephritis, edema of scrotum, and retention of urine belonging to the syndrome of fluid-retention within the body can be treated by the modified recipe.

The recipe is aimed at inducing diuresis, so patients with deficiency of the spleen-qi and with insufficiency of the kidney-qi should ge treated with the recipe in combination with tonics for reinforcing the spleen-qi. It is contraindicated in patients with oliguria due to yin deficiency.

INTERPRETATION

Oriental water plantain rhizome in the recipe is used in large dosage as a principal drug for removing dampness by promoting diuresis. Tuckahoe and Umbellate pore fungus, as diuretics, strengthen the effect of removing excessive fluid and bighead atractylodes rhizome enriches the spleen to transport and transform water and dampness, both being used as assistant drugs. Cassia twig can relieve the exterior syndrome by dispelling pathogenic cold and warm yang to expel qi, acting as an adjuvent drug.

Modern researches have proved that the recipe has the effects of promoting blood circulation and inducing diuresis.

Powder of Ginseng, Poria
and Bighead Atractylodes
(Shen ling bai zhu san)

INGREDIENTS

Semen Nelumbinis	500g
Semen Coicis	500g
Fructus Amomi	500g
Radix Platycodi(stir-baked to deep yellowish)	500g
Semen Dolichoris Album(macerated in ginger juice, bark removed and stir-baked to just dry)	750g
Poria	1000g
Radix Ginseng (stem removed)	1000g
Radix Glycyrrhizae	1000g
Rhizma Atractylodis Macrocephalae	1000g
Rhizoma Dioscoreae	1000g

Decocted in water for oral administration. The dosage can be decided in proportion to the original recipe.

INDICATIONS

Nourishing qi and strengthening the spleen, regulating the stomach and e-liminating dampness. Stagnation of dampness due to deficiency of the spleen marked by lassitude of extremities, general debility, dyspepsia, vomiting or diar-rhea, epigastric distension and fullness, sallow complexion, whitish and greasy coating on the tongue, and feeble and moderate pulse.

In addition, the recipe can be modified to deal with such cases as indiges-tion, chronic gastroenteritis, anemia, nephrotic syndrome, chronic nephritis and other chronic disorders that are ascribable to stagnation of dampness due to defi-ciency of the spleen.

The recipe should be carefully administered to patients with hyperactivity of fire due to yin deficiency; and should be used with discretion by patients associat-ed with deficiency of both qi and yin, or deficiency of yin complicated with defi-ciency of the spleen.

INTERPRETATION

In the recipe, Poria, Ginseng, Licorice root and Bighead atractylodes rhi-zome with mild effect for tonifying qi of the spleen and stomach play together the leading role. White hyaciath bean, Job's-tears, Chinese yam, Lotus seed are ad-ministered to assist Bighead atractylodes rhizome in strengthening the spleen, e-liminating dampness to arrest diarrhea. Amomum fruit, acrid in flavor and warm in property, is used to enliven the spleen by means of aroma to assist the principal drugs in promoting the function of the spleen and stomch, and to arrest vomiting and diarrhea. Platycodon root carries the other drugs in the recipe as-cendingly to reach the upper-warmer for replenishment of the lung.

Modern studies have ascertained that the recipe has the efficacies in regulat-ing gastrointestinal functions, promoting digestion and absorption, arresting di-arrhea, relieving swelling, norishing the organs ans so on.

Prescription for Treating
Diarrhea with Abdominal Pain
(Tong xie yao fang)

INGREDIENTS

Rhizoma Atractylodis Macrocephalae(fried with earth)	12g
Radix Paeoniae Alba	20g
Exocarpium Citri Grandis(fried)	10g
Radix Ledebouriellae	10g

(For cases with prolonged diarrhea, add Rhizoma Cimicifugae 5g).

ACTION

Purging liver-fire and strengthening the spleen; mainly for cases attributive to the suppression of spleen by the stagnated liver-energy, which are manifested as diarrhea with bowel movement upon abdominal pain which is in turn relieved by defecation, increased sounds, thin and white fur on the tongue, wiry and slow pulse.

INDICATION

1. For cases with watery diarrhea, add Radix Puerariae and Semen Plantaginis. For cases with tenesmus, add Semen Arecae and Radix Aucklandiae. For cases with severe abdominal pain, double the dosage of Paeoniae Alba and add Rhizoma Cyperi.

2. Also applicable to cases of chronic enteritis, gastrointestinal neurosis, hyperthyroidism and especially allergic colitis, with frequent diarrhea, attributive to the suppression of spleen by the stagnated liver-energy.

INTERPRETATION

Paeoniae Alba has the effect of calming the liver to relieve abdominal pain, and Atractylodis Macrocephalae has that of strengthening the spleen to eliminate dampness. Two drugs act together to regulate the function of liver and spleen, so-called "inhibiting the wood to help the earth". Ledebouriellae helps the two drugs to release the stagnated liver-energy and activate the spleen-energy. Citri Grandis, after fried, serves to activate the spleen-energy. A good circulation of vital energy may help to relieve pain and a strong spleen may stop diarrhea. A combination of the above four drugs constituents an effective prescription for relieving pain and stopping diarrhea by regulating function of liver spleen.

Pulsatilla Decoction
(Bai tou weng tang)

INGREDIENTS

Radix Pulsatillae	15g
Cortex Phellodendri	12g
Rhizoma Coptidis	6g
Cortex Fraxini	12g

Decocted in water for oral administration.

INDICATIONS

Removing noxious heat and cooling the blood to treat dysentery. Dysentery or diarrhea due to noxious heat marked by more blood and less mucus in stools, abdominal pain, tenesmus, burning sensation in the anus, feverish body, restlessness, thirst with inclination to drink, reddened tongue with yellow coating, and taut and rapid pulse.

The recipe can be modified to treat acute enteritis, bacillary dysentery, amebic dysentery and others which pertain to dysentery of diarrhea due to noxious-heat.

INTERPRETATION

Pulsatilla root plays the role of the principal drug, having the effect of removing noxious-heat from the blood system. Phellodendron bark and coptis root, both bitter in taste and cold in property, can remove noxious-heat and consolidate yin to treat dysentery or diarrhea. Ash bark, with its nature cold and taste bitter and puckery, is used as an astringent to clear away heat and dry dampness, to treat dysentery diarrhea.

Modern researches have confirmed that the recipe has the effects of relieving inflammation, resisting bacteria and ameba, allaying fever, relieving spasm and arresting diarrhea and blood.

Purgative Decoction for
Coordinating the Function of Stomach
(Tiao wei cheng qi tang)

INGREDIENTS

Radix et Rhizoma Rhei	12g
Radix Glycyrrhizae	6g
Natrii Sulfas (infused in)	12g

INDICATIONS

Purging pathogenic heat accumulated in the gastrointestinal tract by laxative action.

Yangming disease marked by gastrointestinal dryness and heat, manifested by obstruction of defecation, thirst and vexation, fever like steaming, abdominal distension and fullness, delirium, yellow tongue coating slippery and rapid pulse as will as eruption, hematemesis, epistaxis, painful swelling of mouth, teeth and throat caused by domination of heat in the intestine and stomach. It can also be indicated for the cases with mild abdominal fullness.

Qi-Regulating Pill of Aucklandia
(Mu xiang shun qi wan)

INGREDIENTS

Radix Aucklandiae

Radix Linderae

Fructus Crataegi

Massa Fermentata Medicinalis

Rhizoma Cyperi

Radix Glycyrrhizae

Fructus Hordei Germinatus

Frictis Aurantii

Poria

Pericarpium Citri Reticulatae Viride

Pericarpium Citri Reticulatae

Semen Arecae

Semen Raphani

Pills, 30g each bottle, 10 bottles per box.

ACTIONS

Relieving stagnation in the chest and regulating qi, strengthening the stomach and promoting digestion.

INDICATIONS

Oppressed feeling in the chest, fullness of abdomen and hypochondrium, poor appetite, dyspepsia. Clinically it may be used to treat the above symptoms in chronic hepatitis, early cirrhosis, chronic gastritis, enteritis, etc.

DIRECTION

To be taken orally with warm boiled water, 6g each time, twice a day.

Contraindicated for patients with weakness, retention of pathogenic heat in the lung and stomach, and for women in pregnancy.

Sophora Powder
(Huai hua san)

INGREDIENTS

Flos Sophorae(parched)	12g
Cacumen Biotae	12g
Spica Schizonepetae	6g
Fructus Aurantii(parched with bran)	6g

Decocted in water for oral administration.

INDICATIONS

Cleaing the bowels to stop bleeding, dispelling pathogenic wind to keep the adverse qi flowing downward. Hemetochezia due to pathogenic wind accumulated in the large intestine marked by bleeding before or after passing stools, or fresh blood in the stools, or dull purplish bloody stools caused by toxic heat in the stomach and large intestine as well as hemorrhoidal bleeding.

Patients with hemorrhoid, colitis and proctopolypus marked by hematochezia caused by pathogenic wind accumulated in the intestine can be treated by the modified recipe.

Drugs in the recipe with cold or cool nature can not be taken for a long time. Patients passing bloody stools without damp-heat are forbidden to the recipe.

INTERPRETATION

Sophora flower, as a principal drug, clears away heat and toxins, cools the blood and removes damp-heat from the large intestine to stop hematochezia. Biota tops removes heat from the blood, eliminates dampness from the large intestine and assists Sophora flower in stopping bleeding; Schizonepeta spike dispels pathogenic wind and stops bleeding. The two drugs mentioned above are assistant drugs. Fruit of citron as an adjuvant and guiding drug, soothes the large intestine to keep the adverse qi flowing downward.

Modern researches have proved that the recipe has the effects of stopping bleeding, relieving inflammation and resisting bacteria.

Stomach Pill of Aucklandia and Amomum Fruit
(Xiang sha yang wei wan)

INGREDIENTS
　　　　Radix Codonopsis Pilosulae
　　　　Rhizoma Atractylodis Macrocephalae
　　　　Pericarpium Citri Reticulatae
　　　　Poria
　　　　Rhizoma Pinelliae Praeparatum
　　　　Fructus Amomi
　　　　Rhizoma Cyperi
　　　　Radix Aucklandiae
　　　　Fructus Aurantii Immaturus
　　　　Fructus Amomi Rotundus
　　　　Herba Agastachis
　　　　Cortex Magnoliae Officinalis
　　　　Radix Glycyrrhizae
Water-paste pills, 1g every 16 pills, 18g per packet.
ACTIONS

Supplementing qi and strengthening the stomach, promoting digestion and stopping vomiting.

INDICATIONS

Dyspepsia due to weakness of the stomach and intestines, manifested as poor appetite, fullness in the stomach, abdominal pain, acid regurgitation, borborygmus, diarrhea and lassitude of limbs.

DIRECTION

To be talen orally with warm boiled water, 9g each time, twice a day.

Uncooked, cold and greasy foods should be avoided.

Stomach-regulating Pill
(Liu he Ding zhong wan)

INGREDIENTS

    Herba Pogostemonis

    Folium Perillae

    Herba Elscholtziae seu Moslae

    Radix Aucklandiae

    Lignum Santali

    Cortex Magnoliae Officinalis

    Fructus Aurantii

    Pericarpium Citri Reticulatae

    Radix Platycodi

    Radix Glycyrrhizae

    Poria

    Fructus Chaenomelis

    Semen Dolichoris Album

    Fructus Crataegi (Stir-roasted)

    Massa Fermentata Medicinalis(Stir-roasted)

    Fructus Hordei Germinatus

    Fructus Oryzae Germinatus

Water-paste pills, 6g per packet.

ACTIONS

Eliminating summer-heat and removing dampness, normalizing the functions of the stomach and spleen, and promoting digestion.

INDICATIONS

For patients affected by summer-heat-dampness and dyspepsia, manifested as chillness, fever, headache, chest tightness, nausea, vomiting, diarrhea and abdominal pain.

DIRECTION

To be taken orally, 3-6g each time, 2-3 times day.

Tangerine Peel and Bamboo Shavings Decoction
(Ju pi zhu ru tang)

INGREDIENTS

Pericarpium Citri Reticulatae	9g
Caulis Bambusae in Taenis	9g
Rhizoma Zingiberis Recens	9g
Radix Ginseng	3g
Radix Glycyrrhizae	6g
Fructus Ziziphi Jujubae	5 pcs

Decocted in water for oral administration.

INDICATIONS

Lowering the adverse flow of qi to relieve vomiting, invigorating qi and clearing away heat. Reversed flow of qi due to weak stomach with heat marked by hiccup, vomiting, anorexia, reddish tongue, feeble and rapid pulse.

Vomiting of pregnancy, incomplete pylorochesis, gastritic vomiting, neurogenic vomiting, ceaseless hiccup after abdominal operation and others marked by the symptoms of reversed flow of qi due to weak stomach with heat can be treated by the modified recipe.

Hicup due to heat of excess type or cold of insuffciency type should not be treated with the recipe.

INTERPRETATION

Tangerine peel regulates the flow of qi, strengthens and normalizes the functions of the stomach and spleen to relieve vomiting. Bamboo shavings clears away stomach-heat to relieve hiccup. The combined use of the two drugs can clear away stomach-heat as well as lower the adverse flow of qi to relieve vomiting. They are both used as principal drugs. Fresh ginger is used to assist the principal drugs in regulating the stomach to arrest vomiting, and combined with Bamboo shavings, achieves the effects of both clearing and warming ao as to prevent the impairment of middle-warmer due to excessive administration of the cold drugs in nature, so they are considered as assistant drugs. Ginseng, licorice root and Chinese-dates, as adjuvant and guiding drugs, invigorate qi, supplement the spleen, regulate the stomach and coordinate the effects of all the other ingredients in the recipe.

Modern studies have proved that the recipe can produce the effects of tranquilizing the mind, relieving inflammation, preventing vomiting and relieving phrenospasm, etc.

Tonic Infusion of Versicolor for Liver
(Yun zhi gan tai chong ji)

INGREDIENTS
Polysaccharidum Versicolor
Medicinal granules(infusion), 10g each packet, 6 packets per box.
ACTIONS
Clearing away pathogenic heat and relieving inflammation, adjusting immunologic function.
INDICATIONS
Chronic active hepatitis, persisting hepatitis, bronchitis, and diseases of hypo-immunologic function.
DIRECTION
To be taken orally, 1 packet each time, 3 times a day.

Two Old Drugs Decoction
(Er chen tang)

INGREDIENTS

Rhizoma Pinelliae	15g
Pericarpium Citri Reticulatae	15g
Poria	9g
Radix Glycyrrhizae Praeparata	3g

Add 3 grams of fresh ginger and a piece of black plum into the above recipe, and then decoct them in water for oral use.

INDICATIONS

Removing dampness to resolve phlegm, and regulating the stomach. Damp-phlegm syndrome marked by cough with profuse whitish sputum, fullness sensation in the chest, nausea, vomiting, dizziness, palpitation, whitish and moist fur of the tongue and slippery pulse.

Bronchitis, gastritis, catarrhal gastritis and other diseases marked by damp-phlegm syndrome can be treated by the modified recipe.

The recipe belongs to pungent and drying prescriptions, therefore, it is contraindicated in Patients suffering from pulmonary tuberculosis with haemoptysis, sticky phlegm due to deficiency of yin and bloody phlegm.

INTERPRETATION

Pinellia tuber, with a pungent flavor and warm and dry nature, is effective in removing dampness to resolve phlegm and lowering the adverse flow of qi and regulating the stomach to arrest vomiting, as a principal drug. Tangerine peel as an assistant drug, with the effect of regulating qi to remove dampness, enables the qi to flow normally and gets the phlegm cleared away. Tuckahoe strengthens the spleen and eliminates dampness; fresh ginger, being able to lower the adverse flow of qi and resolve phlegm, can not only reduce the toxic effect of No. 1 but also strengthen the effects of promoting qi-flow and resolving phlegm of Pinellia tuber and Tangerine peel. A small amount of black plum astringes the lung-qi. The three drugs above are used as adjuvent drugs. Prepared licorice root, as a guiding drug, coordinates the effects of the other drugs, moistens the lung and regulates the stomach.

Modern researches have proved that the recipe has the effects of strengthening the stomach to arrest vomiting, eliminating phlegm to relieve cough and preventing and treating ulcers.

Umbellate Pore Decoction
(Zhu ling tang)

INGREDIENTS

Polyporus Umbellatus	9g
Poria	9g
Rhizoma Alismatis	9g
Colla Corri Asini	9g
Talcum	9g

All the drugs except No. 4 should be decocted in water for oral administration. No. 4 should be taken after being melted by the finished decoction in two separate doses.

INDICATION

Clearing away heat, inducing diuresis and nourishing yin to arrest bleeding. Retention of fluid in the body with impairment of yin due to pathogenic heat marked by difficulty and pain in micturition or blood urine, distention and fullness sensation in the lower abdomen, or insomnia with restlessness, thirst, diarrhea, cough, etc.

Gastroenteritis, mild urinary infection, lithangiuria and nephritis marked by the above syndrome can be treated with the modified recipe.

If the patients have high fever, hyperhidrosis due to excessive pathogenic heat causing severe impairment of yin, the recipe should be used very carefully.

INTERPRETATION

As principal drugs in the recipe, Umbellate pore fungus is sweet, insipid, slightly bitter in taste, with the bitter component able to descend directly to the shaoyin channels, and the sweet and insipid able to remove dampness and induce diuresis; Tuckahoe strengthens the spleen to excrete dampness. Oriental water plantain rhizome, as diuretics, induces diuresis. Talc clears away heat to treat stranguria. Donkey-hide gelatin nourishes yin and moistins dryness to relieve restlessness of deficiency type.

Modern researches have proved that the recipe has antibacterial, antiinflammatory, diuretic and strengthening and tonifying effects.

Universal Relief Decoction for Disinfection
(Pu ji xiao du rin)

INGREDIENTS

Radix Scutellariae(parched with wine)	15g
Rhizoma Coptidis(parched with wine)	15g
Pericarpium Citri Reticulatae(White part removed)	6g
Radix Glycyrrhizae	6g
Radix Scrophulariae	6g
Radix Bupleuri	6g
Radix Platycodi	6g
Fructus Forsythiae	3g
Radix Isatidis	3g
Lasiosphaera Seu Calvatia	3g
Fructus Arctii	3g
Herba Menthae	3g
Bombyx Batryticatus	2g
Rhizoma Cimicifugae	2g

All the above ingredients should be decocted in water for oral administration.

INDICATIONS

Clearing away heat and toxic material, and dispelling wind and other exopathogins.

Infection with swollen head marked by chill and fever, flushed swollen face, heavy eyes, sore throat, dryness of the tongue, thirst, reddened tongue with yellow coating and rapid forceful pulse.

The modified recipe can be used for treatment of diseases with the above symptoms as seen in facial erysipelas, acute parotitis and tonsillitis, carbuncle and other infections swelling in the face.

As the majority of the drugs are bitter and pungent in flavour and cold in nature, patients with yin-deficiency should be cautious when taking this recipe.

INTERPRETATION

In the recipe, Scutellaria root and Coptis root play the role of principal drugs having the effect of dispelling heat-toxin originally affecting the face and head. Being pungent in flavour and cool in nature, Forsythia fruit, Arctium fruit, Peppermint and Batryticated silk worm as assistant drugs in combination, have the effect of dispelling pathoginic wind-heat in the face and head. Licorice root, scrophularia root, Platycodon root and Puff-ball, uaed in combination as adjuvant drugs, have the function of removing heat-toxin from the throat, face and head, they play the part of guiding drugs in combination. Tangerine peel is used to promote the circulation of qi and digestion, cimicifuga rhizome, Bupleurum root to dispel pathogenic wind-heat and to assist the other drugs in reaching the face and head to remove heat pathogens from them.

Modern researches have ascertained that the recipe has the function of relieving inflammation, resisting bacteria and viruses, allaying fever, tranquilizing the mind and alleviating pain.

Yellow Dragon Decoction
(Huang long tang)

INGREDIENTS

Radix et Rhizoma Rhei	10g
Natrii Sulfas (mixed with the decoction)	10g
Radix Angelicae Sinensis	10g
Radix Codonopsis Pilosulae	10g
Fructus Aurantii Immaturus	6g
Cortex Magnoliae Officinalis	6g
Radix Glycyrrhizae	3g
Rhizoma Zingiberis Recens	3 pcs
Fructus Ziziphi Jujubae	3pcs

ACTION

Relaxing the bowels to expel heat evil, invigorating vital energy and nourishing blood; mainly for cases of constipation with occasional watery discharge due to accumulation of heat evil accompanied with deficiency of vital energy and blood, manifested as discharge of thin and foul stools, abdominal pain, trnderness, fever, thirst, tiredness, shortness of breath, dry and yellow fur on the tongue, rapid and weak pulse.

INDICATION

1. By adding Radix Rehmanniae, Radix Ophiopogonis, Radix Scrophulariae and Sea cucumber, and omitting Aurantii Immaturus, Magnoliae Officinalis, Platycodi and Ziziphi Jujubae from this prescription, it is named New Yellow Dragon Decoction. It increases the production of body fluid, relaxes the bowel movement, supports the healthy energy and eliminates the evils, and is indicated for constipation resulting from consumption of body fluid by heat evil, which is accompanied with dry mouth and throat, fatigue, shortness of breath, dry tongue with yellowish or blackish fur, sunken and weak or sunken and unamooth pulse. Yellow Dragon Decoction and New Yellow Dragon Decoction both are purgatives with the action of supporting healthy energy. But the former has a stronger effect of purging heat and is suitable for cases of constipation characterized by overabundance of internal heat evil, while the latter has a stronger effect of nourishing yin and promoting the production of body fluid and is suitable for cases with constipation characterized by consumption of body fluid.

2. Also applicable to cases of bacillary dysentery, amebic dysentery, acute enteritis, typhoid fever, etc. with diarrhea or constipation attributive to hyperactivity of internal heat (or consumption of body fluid by internal heat) accompanied with deficiency of vital energy and blood.

INTERPRETATION

Rhei, Natrii Sulfas, Aurantii Immaturus and Magnoliae Officinalis (the component of Decoction for Potent Purgation) exert a prompt purgative effect to expel the sthenic heat evil accumulated in the intestine and stomach. In order to prevent the exhaustion of vital energy and yin-energy and the occurrence hyperactive heat evil, Angelicae Sinensis and Codonopsis Pilosulae are applied to invigorate the vital energy and blood and support the healthy energy. Platycodi releases the inhibited lung-energy and helps to promote bowel movement. Zingiberis, Ziziphi jujuae and Glycyrrhizae strengthen the stomachenergy and promote the production of vital energy and blood. The prescription, as a whole, aims at purging heat but not impairing the stomach-energy, supporting the healthy energy to eliminate the evils.

Yiguan Decoction
(Yi guan jian)

INGREDIENTS

Radix Rehamanniae(crude)	30g
Radix Adenophorae Strictae	12g
Radix Ophiopogonis	12g
Radix Angelicae Sinensis	12g
Fructus Lycii	12g
Fructus Meliae Toosendan	5g

ACTION

Nourishing the liver and kidney, dispersing the stagnated liver-energy; mainly for the cases of deficiency of liver-yin and kidney-yin, and disorder of liver-energy, which are manifested as chest and hypochondriac pain, acid and bile regurgitation, dry mouth, red tongue, wiry and amall pulse, or hernia, or abdominal mass.

INDICATION

1. For cases with bitter taste and dryness in the mouth attributive to involvement of the stomach by liver-fire, add Rhizoma Coptidis to clear away heat in the liver and stomach; for cases with constipation attributive to deficiency of liver-yin and stomach-yin, add Semen Trichosanthis to lubricate the intestine and promote bowel movement; for cases with spontaneous perspiration attributive to deficiency of liver-yin and kidney-yin, add Cortex Lycii Radicis to clear away the asthenic heat; for cases with abdominal spasmodic pain attributive to imbalance between the function of the liver and spleen, add Radix Paeoniae Alba and Radix Glycyrrhizae to nourish the liver and relive pain.

2. Also applicable to cases of chronic hepatitis, chronic gastritis, cholecystitis, pleuritis, intercostal neuralgia, testitis, etc., manifested as pain over the chest, hypochondrium or lower abdomen, attributive to deficiency of liver-yin and kidney-yin.

INTERPRETATION

Rehmanniae is of sweet flavour and cold nature, which serves to nourish the liver and kidney. Angelicae Sinensis is of acrid flavour and warm nature, which has the effects of tonifying the blood and promoting blood circulation. The combination of these two drugs makes the prescription nourishing but not greasy, acrid but not dry. It not only can nourish the liver, but also can disperse the stagnated liver-energy. Glehniae, Ophiopogonis and Lycii can nourish the liver-yin. Meliae Toosendan can promote vital energy circulation and relieve pain. The combination of the ingredients can nourish liver-yin and let the liver-energy growing freely, so that the corresponding symptoms subside.

Zhuju Pill
(Zhu ju wan)

INGREDIENTS

Rhizoma Coptidis	15g
Rhizoma Zingiberis	6g
Radix Angelicae Sinensis	9g
Corii Asini	9g

ACTION

Clearing away heat, relieving dysentery, warming spleen-yang. nourishing blood and yin; mainly for cases of chronic dysentery with damage of yin-blood, manifested as discharge of bloody and mucous stool, tenesmus fatigue, abdominal pain, anorexia, red and uncoated tongue, sunken, small and rapid pulse, which are at tributive to heat in appearance and cold in body proper, and simultaneous existence of asthenia and sthenia syndrome.

INDICATION

1. Applicable to ulceration of buccal mucosa occurring in infants with malnutrtion, diarhea, dry mouth thirst, red and uncoated tontue, soft and folating, rapid pulse, which is attributive to retaining of dampness-heat evil and damage of spleen-yin.

2. Indicated for cases with foul breath, bitter mouth, dry throat, thirst, restlessness, insomnia, dry stools, red and uncoated tongue, small and rapid

pules, ehich are attributive to deficiency of stomach-yin and hyperactivity of stomach-fire.

3. Also applicabie to cases of chronic bacillary dusemtery and amebicdysentery with damage of yin-blood, or cases of chronic nephritis, duodenitis, infantile indigestion, etc., which are attributive to deficiency of stomach-yin and hyperactivity of stomach-fire, or the retaining of dampness-heat and damage of spleen-yang.

INTERPRETATION

Coptidis acts as the chief drug in the prescription, which clears away heat, dries dampness, eliminates toxic material and relieve dysentery. Zingiberis can warm the spleen-yang and expel dampness. Although the two drugs are different in nature, but they match with each other to purge the evil on one hand and to support the healthy energy on the other hand. Colla Corii Asini can nourish yin-blood when used together with Angelicae sinensis, and fortify yin to relieve dysentery when used together with Coptidis. Angelicae Sinensis used together with Zingiberis can regulate vital energy and blood. In sum, this prescription is indicated chiefly for cases of chronic dysentery when the evil is not eliminated, and yin-blood is consumed and the viscera become cold.

Zuojin bolus
(Zuo jin wan)

INGREDIENTS

Rhizoma Coptidis	12g
Fructus Evodiae	2g

INDICATIONS

Clearing away liver-fire, lowering the adverse rising energy and stopping vomiting; mainly for cases attributive to hyperactivity of fire evil in the liver channel, manifested as hypochondriac pain, eructation, dry mouth, red tongue with yellowish fur, wiry and rapid pulse.

Applicable to cases of diarrhea or dysentery attributive to the attack of dampness-heat evil.

Also applicable to cases of acute gastritis, cholecystitis, bacillary dysentery, allergic colitis, etc. which are attributive to stagnation of liver-fire or attack of dampness-heat.

INTERPRETATION

Coptidis is applied in large dose to purge heart-fire. This is an application of the principle of treating the sthenia-syndrome of mother organ(liver) by purging the child organ(heart) to check the liver-fire. When Evodiae is uaed together with large dose of Coptidis, it serves to disperse the stagnated liver-energy and lower down the adverse rising energy so as to stop vomiting. The two drugs, one cold and one hot, help each other to purge the liver-fire effectively.

图书在版编目（CIP）数据

中医治疗消化系统疾病：英文/侯景伦　赵　昕 编著.-
北京：学苑出版社，1995.10
ISBN 7-5077-0770-9

I.中… II.①侯- ②赵…III.消化系统疾病-中医治疗法-
英文 IV .R259.57

中国版本图书馆 CIP 数据核字(95)第 18121 号

中医治疗消化系统疾病

主　编　侯景伦　赵　昕

学苑出版社出版
（中国北京万寿路西街 11 号）
邮政编码 100036
北京大兴沙窝店印刷厂印刷
中国国际图书贸易总公司发行
（中国北京车公庄西路 35 号）
北京邮政信箱第 399 号　邮政编码 100044
版次：英文版　16 开本　1995 年 10 月第一版第一次印刷
ISBN7-5077-0770-9/R·128

06200
14-E-2942 P